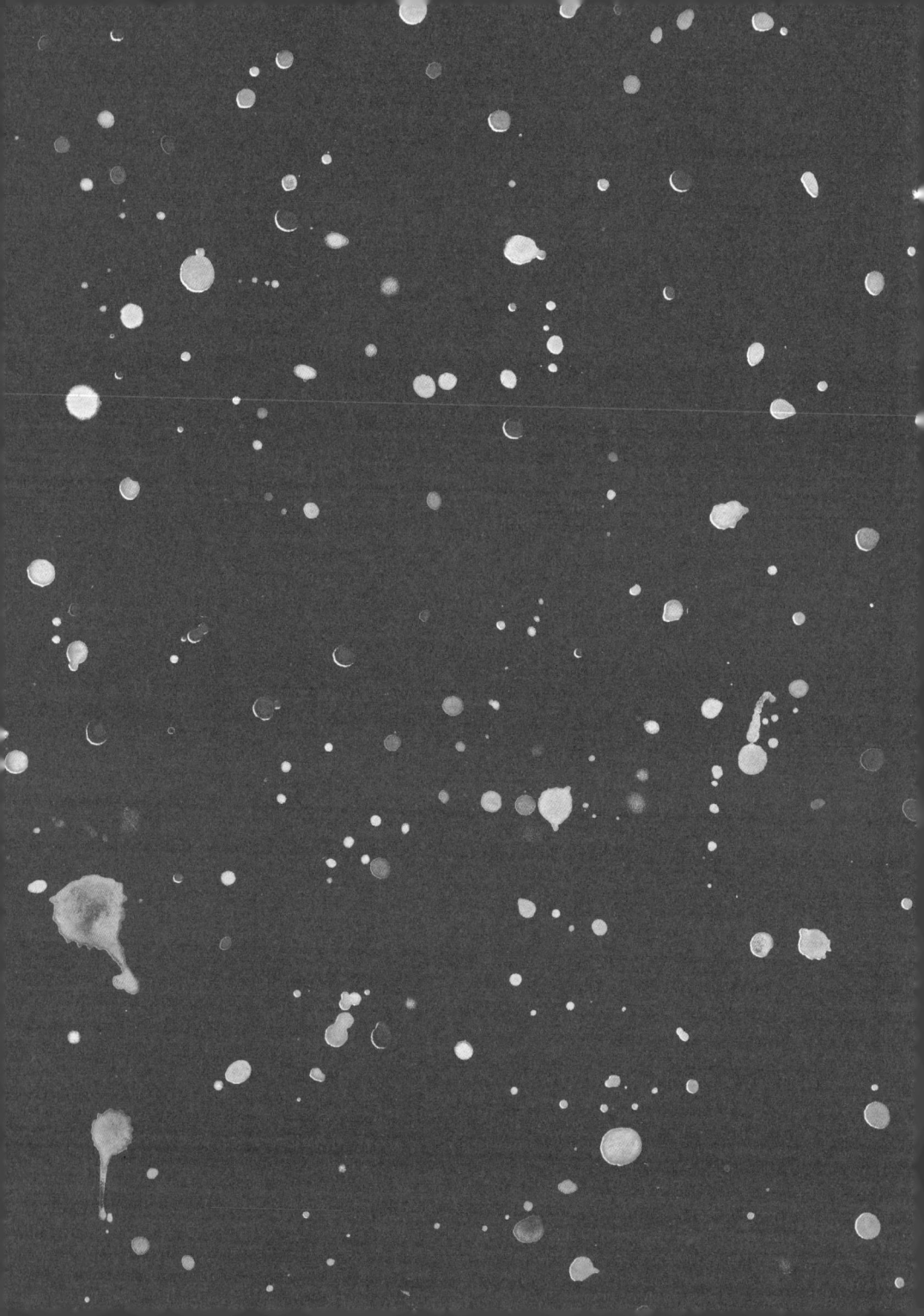

COLD Joy

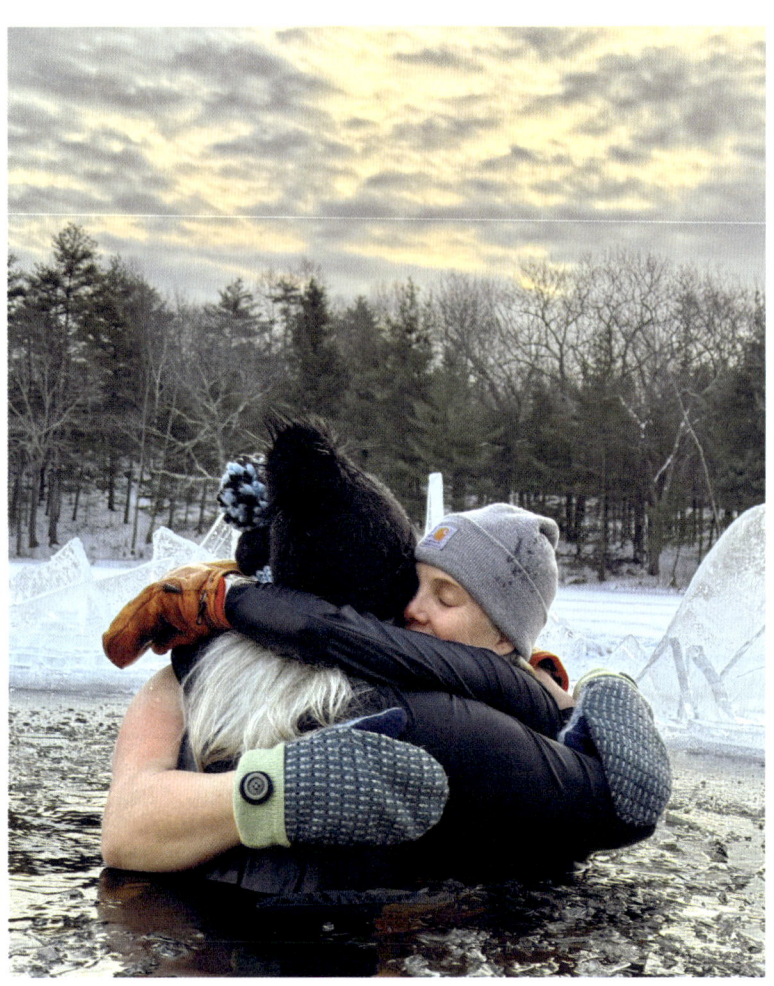

COLD JOY

Experience the Wondrous Power of Cold Water

Libby DeLana
Illustrations by Tjasa Owen

CHRONICLE BOOKS
SAN FRANCISCO

Copyright © 2025 by Libby DeLana.

All rights reserved. No part of this book may be reproduced in any form without written permission from the publisher.

Page 181 constitutes a continuation of the copyright page.

Library of Congress Cataloging-in-Publication Data available.

ISBN 978-1-7972-3529-5

Manufactured in China.

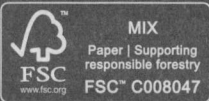

Design by Vanessa Dina.
Typesetting by Frank Brayton.
Illustrations by Tjasa Owen.

This book provides content related to physical and mental well-being. The information contained in this book is presented for educational purposes only. This book is in no way intended as a substitute for the medical advice of physicians. If you seek to use cold plunging to treat a physical and/or mental condition, please consult with your physician or a licensed health-care provider first.

10 9 8 7 6 5 4 3 2 1

Chronicle books and gifts are available at special quantity discounts to corporations, professional associations, literacy programs, and other organizations. For details and discount information, please contact our premiums department at corporatesales@chroniclebooks.com or at 1-800-759-0190.

Chronicle Books LLC
680 Second Street
San Francisco, California 94107
www.chroniclebooks.com

Welcome 7

Chapter One
WONDERING 12

Chapter Two
WADING 28

Chapter Three
WAKING 48

Chapter Four
WITNESS 62

Chapter Five
WILL 78

Chapter Six
WILDNESS 92

Chapter Seven
WELL-BEING 108

Chapter Eight
WAVES 120

Chapter Nine
WISDOM 138

Chapter Ten
WARMTH 152

Reflections 172
Resources 177
Acknowledgments 180
Credits 181
Endnotes 182

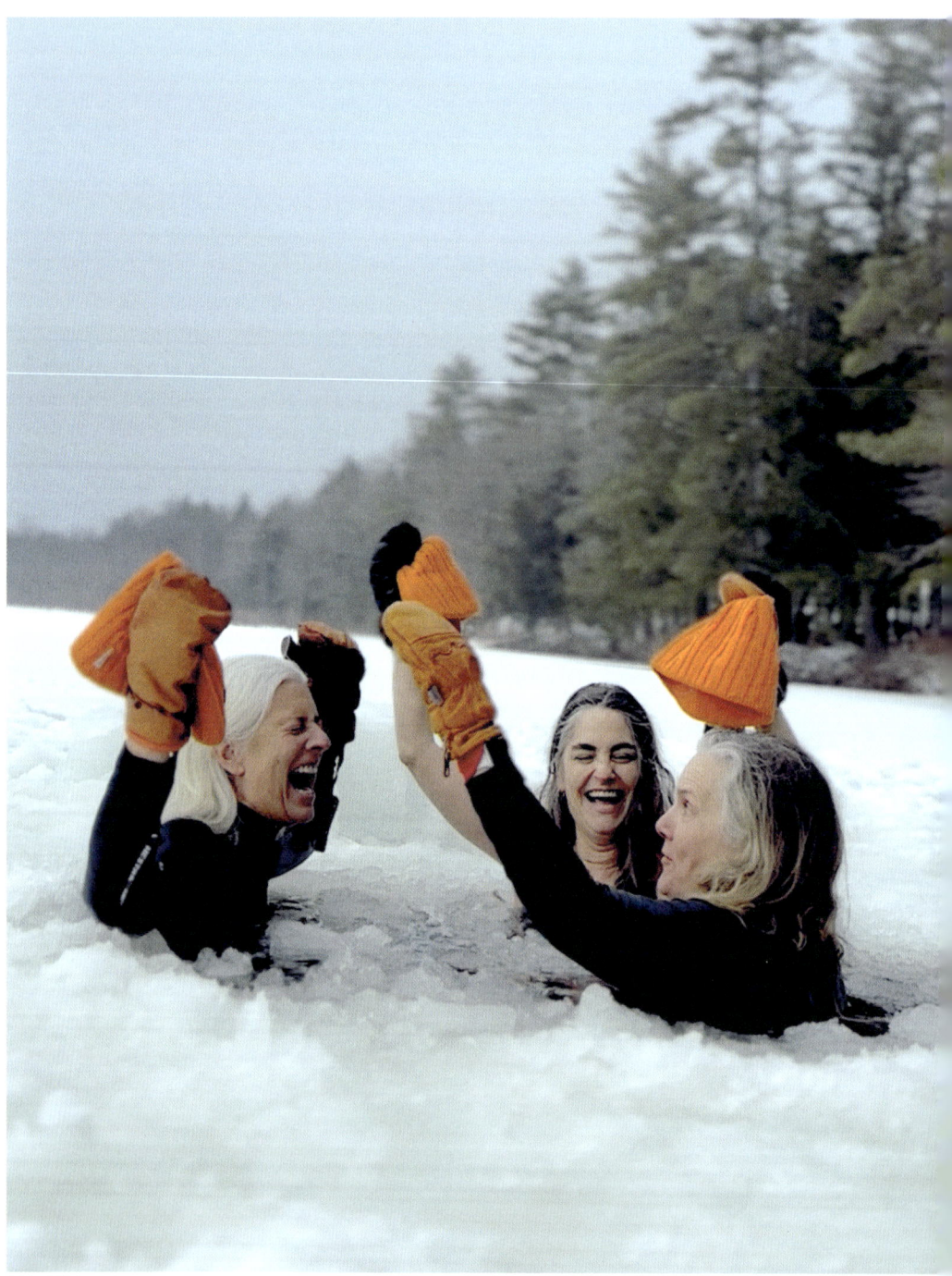

WELCOME

This morning the water felt as though it were reaching for my hand and asking me to dance. The invitation was made with so much kindness and care, I was almost too bashful to accept it. Steam curled from the water's surface in long, elegant fingers, and the sun glanced from the tops of the waves, flickering silver. The night heron, hunched over but glorious, watched from the reeds, which chattered with morning breeze, one of the last warm winds of the year.

"Won't you come in?" the water said, rolling onto the beach, depositing vacant shells and pebbles—strange but perfect gifts—at my toes.

I waited for a moment. She reached for me again, and this time, I reached back, walking in up to my middle, letting her hold me, move me, love me.

For the past five years, I have started most of my days dancing this dance with the cold water. It is ritually significant to me, an expression of self-love, earth-love, spirit-love, people-love. The water is my partner, my guide, my classroom, and my playground. It is truly a comfort to me.

But cold water is *un*comfortable, isn't it?

Just the thought of an icy river or unheated swimming pool elicits a physical reaction—shivers, cringes, walls going up, alarms going off, held breath. I have richly painted childhood memories of this feeling, standing on an old gray dock with a Speedo-clad gaggle, our toes curled around the precipice, bargaining with one another, "You go first," "No, you go first." All of us tense, our hands balled into fists and our faces crumpled.

Eventually someone—usually not me—would jump in. There would be shrieks and splashes, then joy and fun. The rest of us would follow. The first several seconds were indeed uncomfortable, but on the other side was jubilation. To me, cold-water immersion is about making jubilation into a habit. It is about cold joy, champagne sparkles, and the feeling of spinning—dancing a dance that, over time, we've forgotten we know. So, every morning, when the water asks, I walk into her arms and let her lead.

Cold Joy is about accepting invitations, staying open to change, allowing our stories as humans to unfold slowly, and finding the courage to question false narratives. Like many devotees, when I first saw people online sinking chin deep into their icy tubs, I said, "Never."

But over time a quieter, wiser, more-curious voice has emerged, asking *"Why not?"*

This book is my journey to that question and many, many more beyond it. It is a record of what cold immersion can reveal in us, how it can teach us, guiding us to lessons about ourselves and the world that we may not find otherwise, huddled so close to the cozy hearth of daily life. I take you from the initial wonderings about cold dipping, into the water, and on to a deeper practice, sharing the challenges that have come up for me along the way and the tools that have helped me nourish and sustain the best damn habit I've ever had. Together, we'll go to wild places. Sometimes, they'll be swirling rivers that lead to the ocean, other times they'll be eddying pools inside us. Some days, we'll climb unclimbable walls, other days we'll smile and wave to the harbor seals.

If you're looking for a medical argument for cold immersion, or any argument really, you won't find it in these pages. This is cold immersion through a loving, heart-forward lens, centered on my own experience, our relationship with water through history, and the stories generously shared with me by others. I am not a doctor, and even if I were, data on the long-term effects of cold exposure is still very much emerging. Many of the possible benefits are overstated by enthusiasts, while the very real risks don't make the highlight reels. It is important for every person interested in the practice to consult with a trusted medical provider.

Also—and I know this may disappoint some—I won't be spouting definitive instructions. The best version of this practice for me might not be the best for you, and that's perfectly fine! What I can and will extend to you is an invitation—to personal growth, deeper inquiry, joy, and learning to dance your dance all over again.

Let's get in the water.
What's the best
that could happen?

CHAPTER ONE

WOND

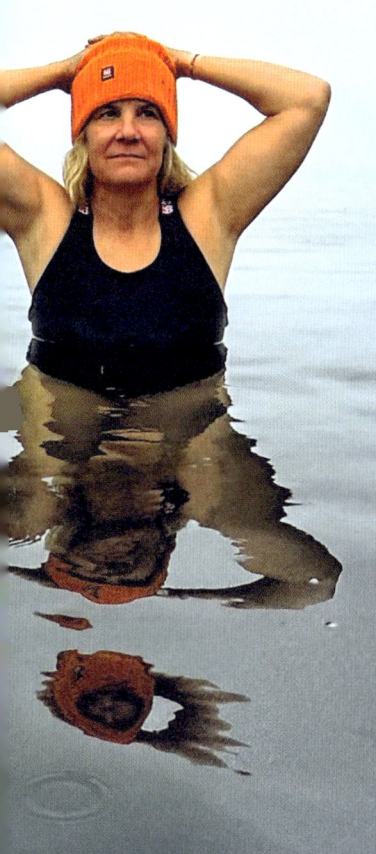

ERING

Camp Treetops was a renegade summer program burrowed in the brightest green parts of the Adirondack Mountains, surrounded by hardwood forests and singing rivers. I attended for several years in the 1970s, in my early teens. I was proud to be there. The kids at Treetops loved the outdoors—we were tough, we weren't afraid to get our socks dirty. We slept in lean-tos, attended to barn chores, picked our dinner from the garden, and went on hiking excursions that lasted days. We were a fierce and fly-bitten bunch, carrying our knives and tin cups up the side of Mount Van Hoevenberg and Owls Head Mountain, along the shores of Saranac Lake. These were our glorious days, drinking nature through our noses and smacking mosquitoes from each other's shoulders. I wasn't just comfortable on the trail, I was at home.

The daytime temps were blissful, in the mid-seventies, but at night they could creep closer to fifty. This wasn't extreme, especially for our fire-making, trail-blazing lot, except for once, when it was. One night, with my sleeping bag pulled up to my earlobes, I couldn't get warm. I rubbed my feet together and stuffed my hands in my pockets, but I was chilled through. Nothing helped. I knew what I should do—wake a counselor, cuddle up with a friend, make some tea, ask for help—but I was too embarrassed, too shy, too "thirteen." I shivered all night, scared and miserable. I felt unsafe, maybe for the first time in my (very lucky) life.

I woke up the next morning viscerally afraid of the cold and I stayed that way well into adulthood. I was the one who complained about the office air-conditioning in her puffer jacket and beanie. I was the one who couldn't make the trip up north because of an invented "prior commitment." I was the reason dear friends kept extra sweaters and mitts in their trunk. Until just a few years ago, I defined myself as someone who *hated* the cold. So many of us define ourselves that way.

Our relationship with the cold is complicated. We bundle up, crank the heat, fly south like birds and butterflies for the winter. Our lore is filled with sinister ice queens, whipping winds, and blinding blizzards. Even our language around the cold is vilifying: When we're "given the cold shoulder," we've been ostracized. When we're "out cold," we've lost consciousness. We *escape* the cold whereas we *keep* warm, hoarding it like a resource. When I tell people that I start my day by spending several minutes up to my shoulders in 40-something degree water, some actually *recoil*, physically leaning away from, not into, the conversation. My reaction used to be similar. I bristled at the idea of cold water, body tightened and mind closed. But the more I opened up, the less true my negative associations with cold seemed to be. Openness became curiosity, curiosity became courage, and courage became a transformative, transcendent cold-immersion practice. My story is different now. Cold is inviting and awakening. Cold is a teacher and a friend. It has been a steady companion, a precious gift, a truth-teller, and an agent of change.

I believe many of us have a formative, traumatic experience like mine, an experience that transformed "cold" into "danger," "loneliness," "numbness," or "death," even. I don't believe these stories are wrong. Cold exposure *is* vulnerable, it *is* uncomfortable, and it can indeed be isolating. The problem with these stories is they're incomplete. If we stay open, mustering the patience and wonder to endure, to turn the next page and the next, our narrative can change and, magically, we can too. For me, cold exposure is less about the cold and more about exposure. Hidden in cold water, the great mystery of ourselves is waiting to be revealed.

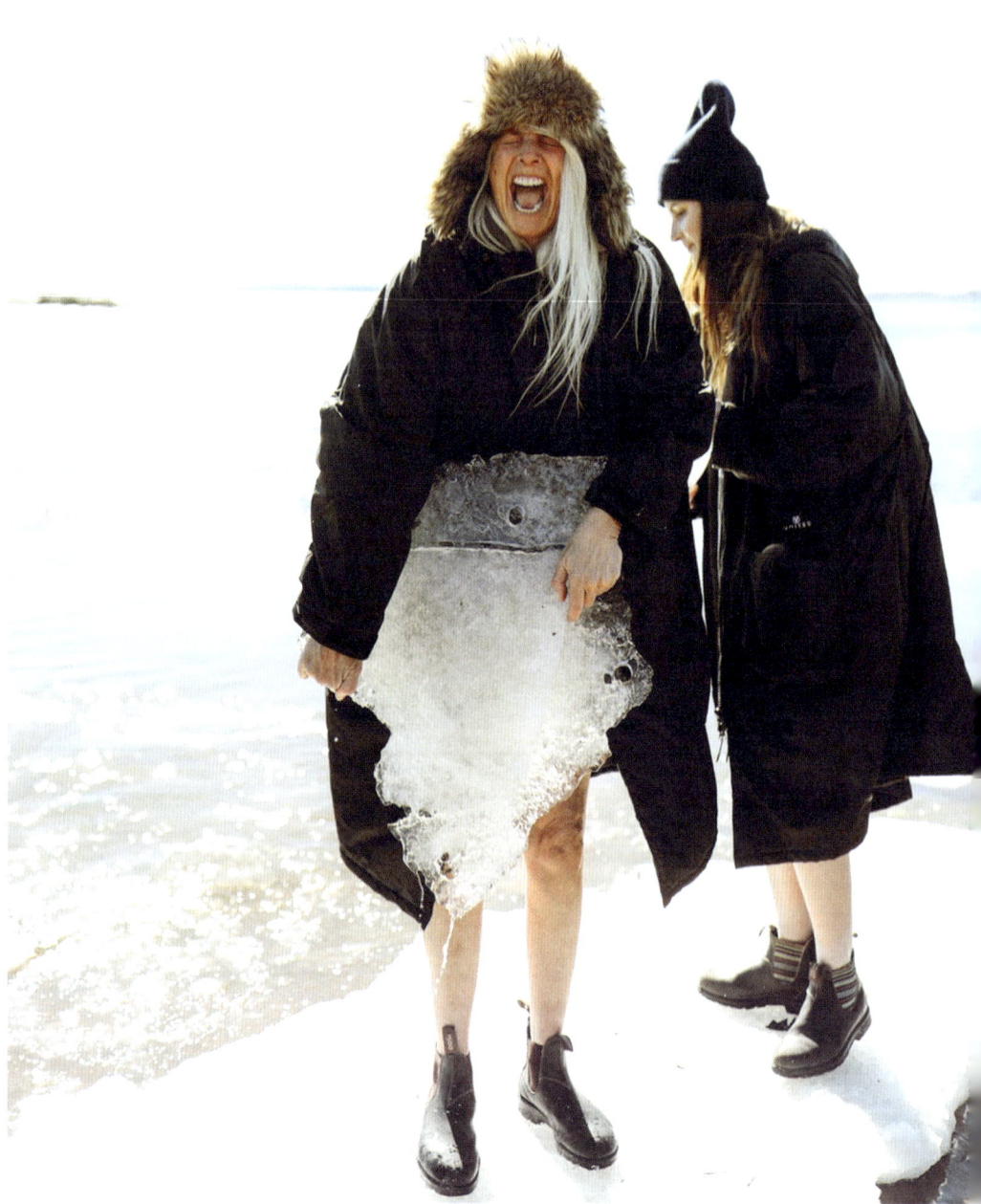

OLD
COLD

Today we like to wear our winter jackets to the movies and shuffle around our climate-controlled houses flannel pajama-ed and cozy slipper-ed (dedicated cozy slipper shuffler over here;). We put an awful lot of layers between us and the cold, but it hasn't always been this way.

For thousands of years, across countless cultures, cold water has been a cornerstone of physical and spiritual health. For most of our history, we've loved the cold, or at the very least, understood it as something of value. The earliest mentions of cold exposure date back as far as 3500 BCE and echo through the ages in a multitude of medical, cultural, and social practices. From Hua Tuo to Hippocrates, the Roman baths to the Finnish saunas, the cold has been an important part of how people heal, how we live, and who we are. But somewhere along the way, something in our collective consciousness shifted, *our* story changed.

Technology, even in its most basic forms, has made our world more comfortable. We have our warm woolly sweaters now and can make dinner in the microwave. We drive through our days instead of walk. Our children have indoor recess whenever the temperature drops below freezing. Much of our innovation has been centered around making life easier and more efficient, but not necessarily better. We simply aren't exposed to extreme cold (or heat) anymore. We may not even know what it feels like. Something that for many cultures was once an inevitability of daily life is now an anomaly. We are not *unable* to be uncomfortable though, and many of us forget that. We have more resilience, focus, and fortitude than we're able to see from the comfortable confines of modern life. To experience our full strength, we need to test it. To see our full selves, we need to get vulnerable. To get over our fear of cold water, we need to get in.

I don't think of immersion as doing something new with my body, I think of it as returning something to it that got lost along the way. I think of cold exposure as a way of telling my story, all the way through.

NEW COLD

Cold is undeniably hot right now. It's been a boon to body-hacking podcasters, an emerging area of scientific study, and a full-blown social media sensation. There's a lot to be curious about and, of course, there are many points of contention too.

There are countless opinions surrounding what defines a cold-exposure practice and what kind of practice is best. Some, like the incredibly popular Wim Hof Method, emphasize breathwork, willpower, and physical wellness. Others, like contrast therapy, employ alternating exposures of heat and cold. There are people who practice cold swimming and others who simply turn the faucet to C after shampooing their hair. There are people who are very particular about water temperature, duration of exposure, and how they measure their success. And there are people (like me) who hardly think of those things at all.

We also come to cold water for vastly different reasons. Many people, if not most, are intrigued by the possible health benefits and the physical test a cold plunge provides. My practice is rooted in feeling over function. I am learning myself—exploring and challenging my identity—through cold water. I am also learning my world, becoming a little more connected to nature and aware of my role in our ecosystem. For me, exposure looks like regular immersion in cold water that brings calm to my mind and body. Sometimes, I hop into the Merrimack River, other times, I use a stock tank in my backyard. There is no set time or temperature, though anything above 60 degrees tends to be a little balmy for me, and temps teetering close to freezing are generally not advisable.

LESSON: "The Mermaid Method"

My practice, like water itself, is fluid, but invariably, follows these basic tenets:

PERSONAL: More important than **how** I practice, is **why**. I'm coming to water with questions about myself. I feel a deep desire to immerse and emerge. I am in conversation with myself, not competition.

POWERFUL: This practice is changing the way I feel in my mind and body. Beyond the typical metrics, I feel that I'm growing. My understanding for myself and my world is expanding.

PRACTICAL: I can continue my practice regularly and safely, without duress. Getting in the water makes my time out of the water better, easier, and more enjoyable.

The water is tender, joyful, insightful, generous, and wise. The water holds all our stories, our wisdom, sweat, and tears. In a very successful practice, I **feel** held. If I have one hope for the cold-curious, it's that the water tells you a more complete story about who you are.

THE LAST DROP

Before I began this cold-exposure practice, I made a lot of choices about the kind of person I was and the things I was (and wasn't) capable of. Cold exposure has taught me that my great story is still unfolding, and that my nature is a matter of discovery, not decision-making. I'll probably never forget the tautness of my sleeping bag around my shoulders as I hugged my spindly thirteen-year-old legs into my chest, but I know now it was a small chapter in a big life. I'll also never forget the gentleness of the cold wrapping herself around me when I first got into the water, and the wonderful songs the ocean sang that morning.

WATERWORLD

Cold exposure might seem like the (literal) cool new thing, but our tradition with cold goes back far **and** wide. Here's a quick look at a few places in history it popped up:

3500 BCE, ANCIENT EGYPT: Several mentions of cryotherapy as a healing agent appear in *The Edwin Smith Papyrus*, perhaps the oldest medical text in existence!

4TH CENTURY BCE, GREECE: Hippocrates suggests cold as an effective analgesic in his theory of the "four humours."

6TH-8TH CENTURY CE, JAPAN: Misogi, or cold meditation practices, develop alongside other Shinto purification traditions.

14TH-15TH CENTURY CE, INDIA: The *Padma Purana*, a Hindu text, is composed, containing references to ritual cold bathing and ayurvedic water traditions.

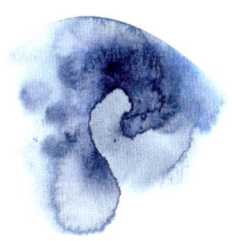

WATERWORLD cont'd

70 CE, ANCIENT ROME: Bath culture emerges. A "frigidarium" is included as one of the three main chambers of a conventional bathhouse.

1600 CE, RUSSIA: Cold swimming becomes part of the Epiphany tradition, though cold swimming may have been practiced in Russia as far back as pagan times.

1697 CE, ENGLAND: Physician John Floyer publishes *An Enquiry into the Right Use and Abuses of the Hot, Cold, and Temperate Baths in England*, recommending a "cold regimen" for optimal health.

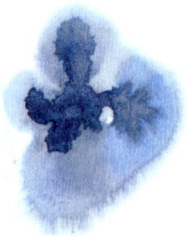

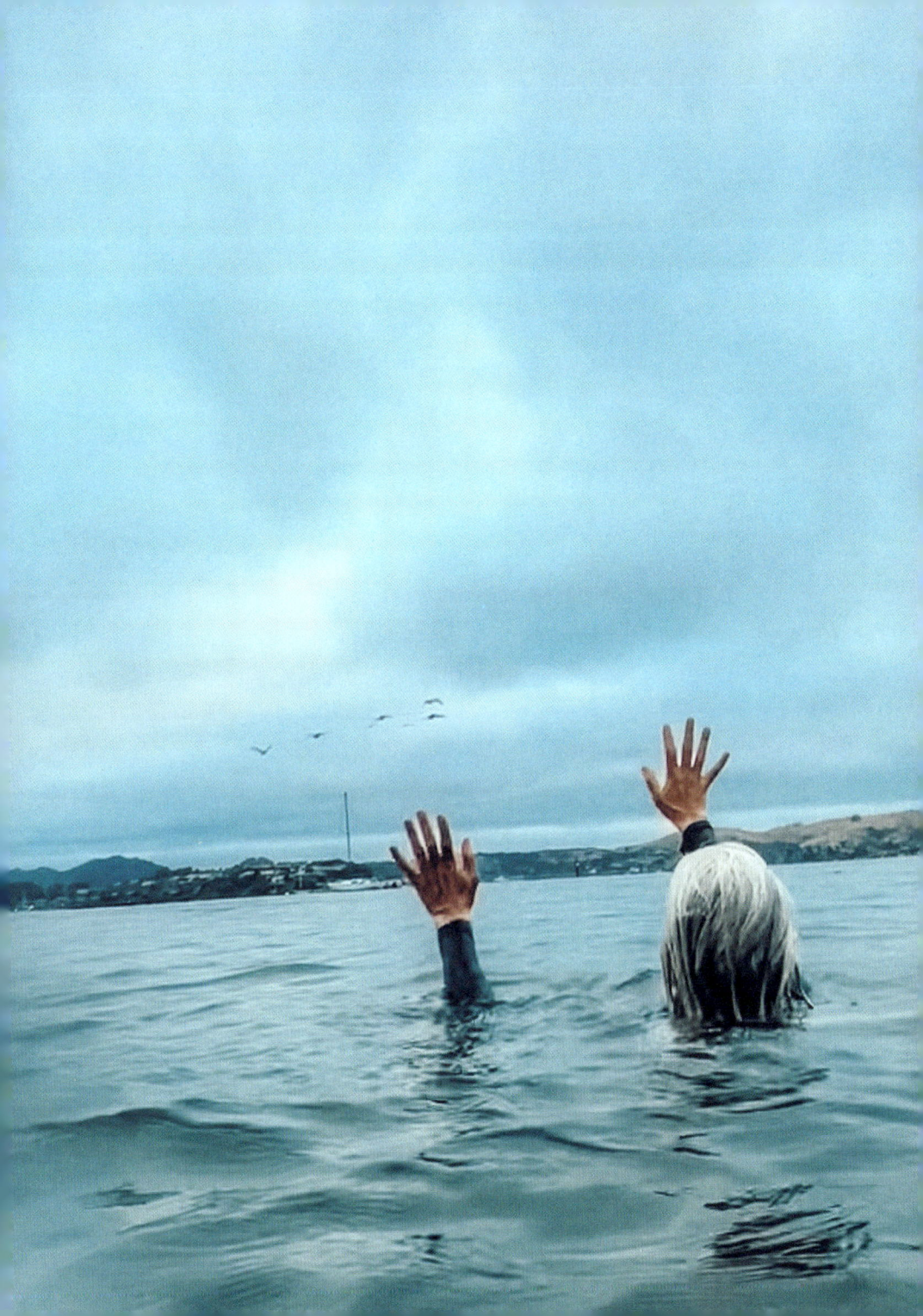

A SPLASH OF SCIENCE

While data is still emerging, many scientists (thank you Dr. Susanna Søberg) and medical researchers are riding the cold-exposure wave along with us and studying the benefits of immersion practices. There's a long way to go, but early research is promising and suggests that cold water *may*:

- Increase the activity of the sympathetic nervous system, potentially improving alertness and responsiveness.

- Reduce insulin resistance and boost insulin sensitivity, regulating blood sugar.

- Activate brown adipose tissue (brown fat) and increase metabolism.

- Increase plasma noradrenaline concentrations by up to 530 percent and dopamine by 250 percent, improving cognitive function and mood.

- Lower cortisol levels and decrease stress.

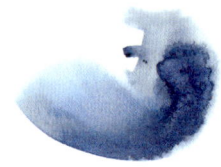

I'll never forget the
gentleness of the cold
wrapping herself around
me when I first got into
the water, and the wonderful
songs the ocean sang
that morning.

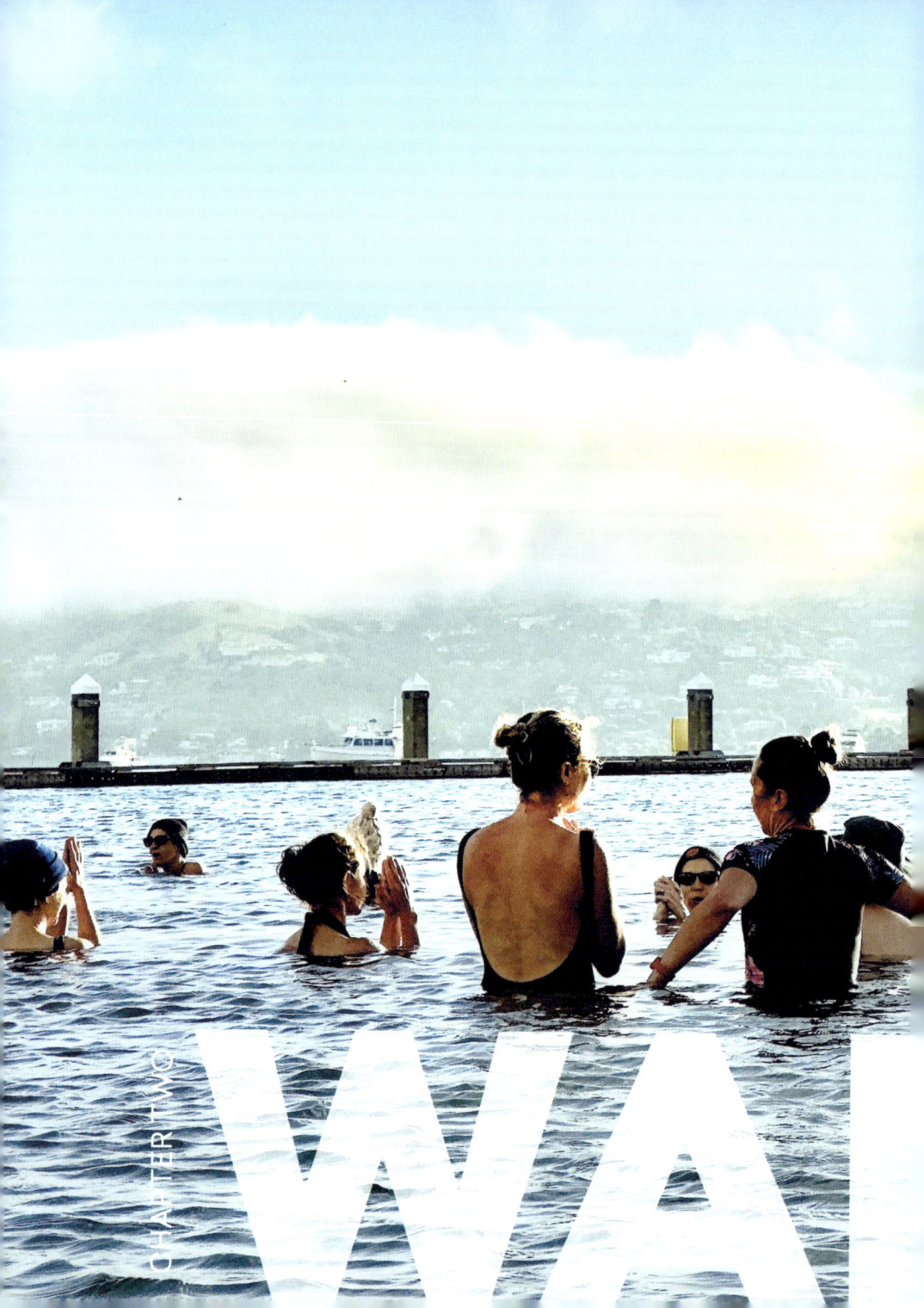

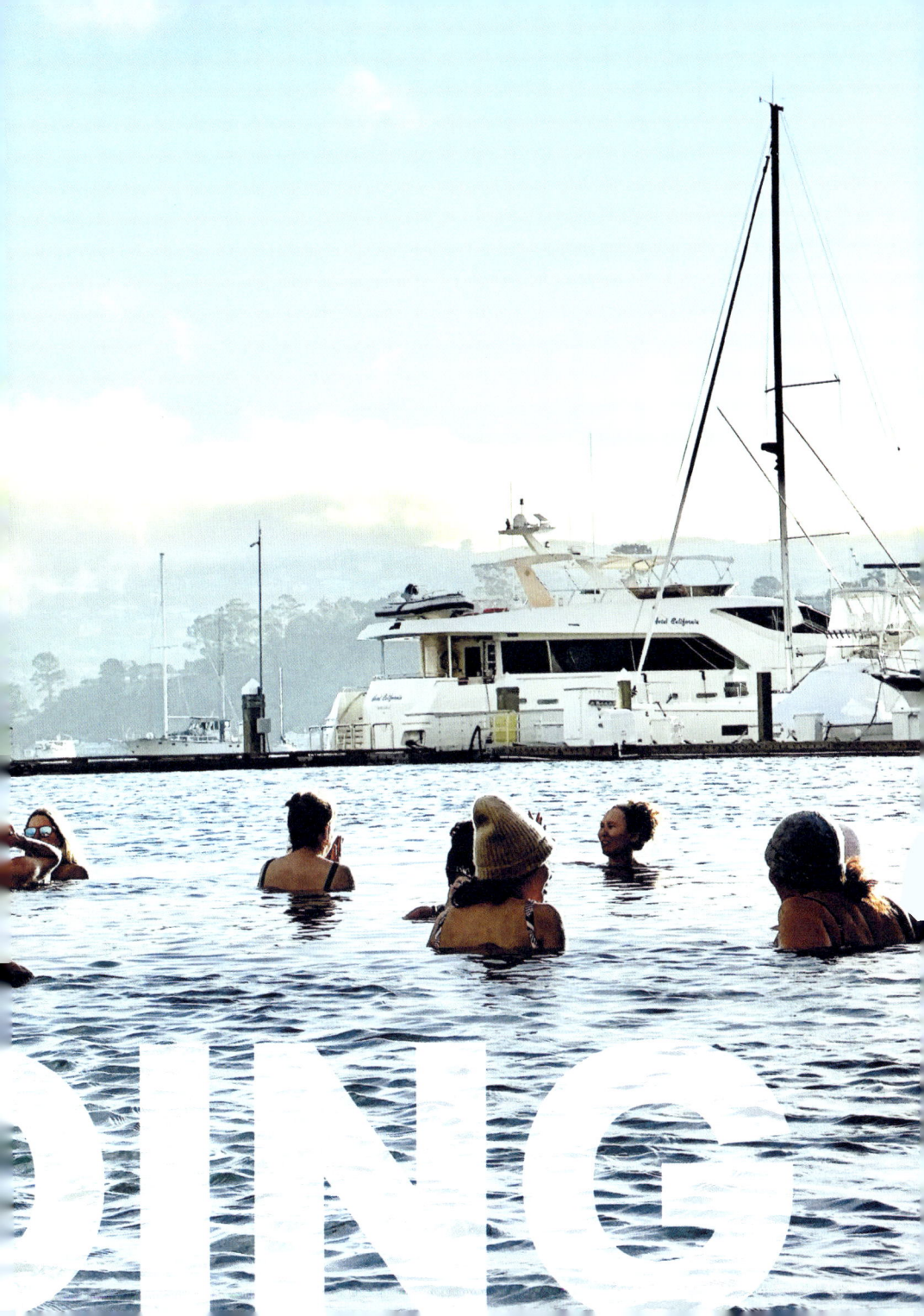

The snowy owls came early in 2020, flying to Newburyport in November, as opposed to the usual January. In the middle of a pandemic, the premature arrival of the owls was hardly a seismic shift, but I noticed them: salt-and-pepper wings tucked under their bodies, basking, I suppose, in the warmth of a Massachusetts winter. The entire world was in flux, along with the owls, along with me.

Truthfully, the disruption in my life extended far beyond a new routine of masking up, locking down, and sanitizing my green beans. Nothing wakes us up, shakes us up, like a glimpse of our mortality. People got new puppies and families shifted. Sourdough bakers were born and beloveds buried. One change made another and another and another. My marriage dissolved. My boys grew up (over the course of an afternoon, I swear!). A long and fruitful professional relationship also came to an end. As everything around me changed course, I wondered if I could too. The thought thrilled and terrified me.

For years, I'd started my days with a morning walk. During quarantine, my fabulous "Pod Squad"—Cheryl, Beth, Will, and Orren, my son—joined in. In the days of isolation, a walk together felt celebratory, jubilant, and, at times, deliciously rebellious. The world was on fire, but we fought back, strolling with mugs of warm tea. We often met at Plum Island, a barrier isle with a magical stretch of beach just past Cape Ann. It's staggeringly gorgeous, the capital city of my heart. When it rains there, you can see purple garnet streaked through the sand. Piping plovers nest on the beach, hidden in the brown grasses. Seals stop by to say hello, rolling their bodies through the water, always smiling.

I loved walking near the water, but I never went in. The ocean had the allure of a forbidden room in a big house, only to be used by grown-ups, on grown-up occasions. I took pictures of the water, listened to its latest music, and observed it. Some days it was calm and others raging. Some days it was leaf green and others it was so clear you could count pebbles at the bottom. I admired its fluidity. We would walk and talk and pause, gazing at the sea, imagining what it would be like to be so mutable and changeable, so wild and free.

On a day that was gray but bright, clouds backlit with the promise of sun, we took our usual walk at our usual beach. Midway through, we stopped, looked at each other, and stripped down, full of bravado, chai, and not a lot of common sense. The moment was serendipitous, exquisitely giggly and liberating. It felt like *mine*.

When the water first held me, it was like someone flipped on a light switch. It was a shock of sensation—aching, yearning, screaming, laughing, potently curious, joyful, zany. The water was dark and frigid, but my senses were sharp—sparkly bright. I felt my body absorb the energy of the sea, which that day was more playful than calming. We were in for only a few seconds, but I knew there was something eternal about what I had experienced. I had changed. I *could* change. I *was* wild, free, and happy. And I loved that about myself. In fourteen seconds, the water and these people had taught me things I'd been trying to learn for years.

Skin goosebump-y, clouds of breath escaping our noses, we stood on the beach afterward in disbelief, trembling, clumsily trying to stuff our sticky wet bodies into our even stickier dry clothes. Back in the car, I sat alert and dazzled by the cold water. I was alive again and in love, not just with the water but also with these people and with me. There is nothing else like your first dip.

DIP VERSUS PLUNGE

From a distance, a cold-exposure practice can seem more extreme than enlivening. And truly, when you submerge to your neck for the first time, it may feel like a free fall. You might shriek, laugh, cry, or become momentarily breathless. You might jump right out (and that's OK!). But cold exposure isn't a contest of strength or stamina; the challenge is in self-compassion, body awareness, moving beyond external pressure to internal wisdom. In our age of internet adrenaline junkies and wellness fads, I think it's important to make this distinction. Attitude is everything. And words matter!

I rarely refer to my immersion as a cold *plunge*. Something about the language feels severe and almost dangerous, the exact opposite of what a healthy, sustainable practice should be. Early on, I heard someone refer to it as a dip (I think it was Kath of @redhotchillydippers), so I adopted this language too. The term simply feels more loving to me. It conveys a sense of refreshment and relief that aligns with my goals. I urge others to consider this reframe, especially when they're just starting out or determining if the practice is right for them. And it isn't right for everyone.

If you're looking to push your body to the extreme, lose weight, pry open your identity, and start rearranging the cupboards, consistent practice will not scratch the itch for long. If you can commit to patience, gentleness, and exploration—more of a blooming than a bashing-the-door-in—then we're in business.

The water's cold, let's jump in!

LESSON:

Ready, Set, Go!

Before You Dip

Romantic as it can be, running headlong into the Atlantic Ocean, full of piss and vinegar, is not the best way to begin your cold-water journey. Any new practice should be taken on with a lot of thought and humility, especially one that could put your health and safety at risk. Here are a few steps you can take before diving in.

TALK TO YOUR DOCTOR: Though cold exposure has been around roughly as long as we've been keeping time, research into the risks and benefits is just beginning. Not much is known about the long-term effects, good or bad. We do know it isn't safe for some people. Speak with your healthcare providers about whether or not immersion is a good fit for you and make it a part of an ongoing conversation with them.

TALK TO YOUR PEOPLE: Aside from the physical risks of cold exposure, there are also practical safety considerations. When starting, you should never dip alone, especially in the open or deep water. Even if you're at home, best practice is to have someone around in case of an emergency. Always keep your charged phone nearby. Learn the signs of hypothermia—they can include numbness, confusion, irregular breathing or heartbeat, slurring speech, and shivering—and consider what those may look like in others. Before you dip, have a plan for after to get warm and dry. Always get in feet first and never dip if you're not feeling well or if you're under the influence of alcohol.

I do love a hot toddy (or a not toddy) when I'm all done and dried though.

TALK TO YOURSELF: Before every dip, I like to check in with myself. I take inventory of how I'm feeling physically and emotionally. I commit to listening to my body and looking out for myself and those around me. Some questions that come up frequently are: How did I sleep last night? How am I feeling physically? Am I dehydrated? Am I sad or angry? Am I going to try to push through something I shouldn't?

Answers to those questions invariably impact the way I come to the water. If I didn't sleep well, the shock of the cold water may be more intense. If I'm upset, I may need to remind myself to breathe. If I can't go to the water honestly, I don't go at all. There's no shame in trying again another time.

Pay attention to what your body is saying in the water. If anything feels off during your practice, stop immediately and let your doctor know. Commit to going slowly so that you can properly observe yourself. Keep notes. I have a water journal.

What to Bring

One of the best things about cold exposure is all the stuff you **don't** need. You don't have to buy a pricey ice bath machine. If you've got wild water nearby, you don't even need plumbing. If you're dipping indoors (or in Europe!) you may not even need a swimsuit.

For a basic shower, tub, pool, or outdoor dip in moderate weather you need:

- **Water: This can be in a rubber basin or stock tank filled up with your garden hose, a shower, a pool, or the sea.**
- **A swimsuit (or not, if you're cheeky)**
- **An old bathmat for the ground, and a towel for the body**
- **Warmies for after. I love a Voited swim coat and a secondhand wool sweater.**
- **A fully charged cell phone**
- **A buddy to cheer you on**
- **A first aid kit**
- **Ice is nice but isn't necessary for first-timers.**

How to Get In

"What does it feel like?"

I get this question more than any other, and while I don't believe I can answer it for another person in another body, I love sharing what I feel during a typical dip:

ELECTRICITY: When I first get into the water, a wave of energy charges through my body. Sometimes this feels achy or like a full-body pinch. I don't want to get your hopes up, but the sensation can even be a little ticklish. I normally get in first thing in the morning and submerge quickly, up to my neck. I don't wait. I get in right away. It doesn't get warmer waiting.

Try to stay present in this moment, feel it all the way in. Breathe. Breathe. Breathe.

EUPHORIA: After the first fifteen seconds or so my body relaxes into the water. The initial shock softens into what is often a giggle fit. I might get an ice cream headache in my elbows or feel magic in my toes. Most days, I'm smiling.

It takes immense focus to get to this lovely, silly feeling. Celebrate it. Good luck **not** celebrating it. Give it up for you!

EASE: My breathing is steady and deep, no longer labored. I get to calm (more on this later). I am acutely aware and very peaceful.

Sit in this peace, enjoy it, take it with you when you go.

EXPANSION: I feel a comfortable sense of completion. My mind may drift out of the water and begin its day. When it does, I know it's time to go.

You did it! Get out slowly and keep listening to your body. Emerging is often the hardest part. Say thank you to the water and to yourself.

THE LAST DROP

A healthy, conscious cold-water practice comes from a place of self-love, not a desire for self-improvement. The goal isn't to become someone else, it's to discover more of yourself. I often return to that morning at Plum Island with the plovers and the magic sky and the swirling laughter of my loved ones. The feeling of the butterflies is still there, alive and well in my belly.

In the moment, I thought it was courage that sent me running off into the surf like a wild woman, but it was something bigger than being brave. Now I look back at that first dip (and all my dips since) as an act of curiosity, love, deep listening, trust in my community, and radical self-compassion.

TAKING THE TEMPERATURE WITH YOUR HEALTHCARE TEAM

Though it might not be a roaring good time, talking with your doctor is crucial before beginning your practice. Here are a few guidelines I use to shape my discussion:

BE SPECIFIC. Let your doctor know exactly what you plan to do. There's a big difference between a fifteen second, 68°F shower and swimming Lake Michigan in February (both can be fabulous!). The more information you have, the more tailored the advice your provider can give.

BE HONEST. Make sure your doctor has your complete health history, a clear picture of how your body feels **right now**, and the lifestyle you lead. Don't fudge the details; your doctor is a human too. Cold exposure is not safe for everyone, and you want to be sure you can walk into the practice confidently.

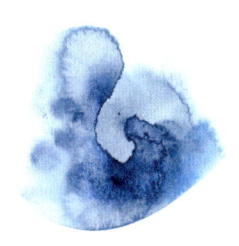

TAKING THE TEMPERATURE WITH YOUR HEALTHCARE TEAM cont'd

BE A PEST. Even if you get the green light, **keep talking** about your practice with your doctor. If a question comes up, ask. If you're worried about something, bring it up. Be vigilant in reporting (and recording) physical changes.

KINDS OF COLD

Reader, if variety is the spice of your life, rest assured there are lots of different ways to get wet. Here are the most popular ways to do it:

SHOWER POWER: Turning the faucet to cold at the end of your shower is an awesome (and practical) way to ease into cold exposure, build tolerance, and see how your body reacts.

POOL PARTY: The shallow end of an unheated pool is great for a group dip. It may get too warm during the warmer months, but when the air is cold, pool temps can be just right.

TUB TIME: Whether it's a stock tank or a space-age ice bath, a basin creates a convenient, controlled, dedicated space for your practice. Be sure to keep it clean and covered, skim out the yuckies, and drain and refill when needed. I change the water in my tank every few weeks, that's it.

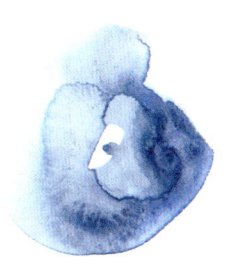

KINDS OF COLD cont'd

WILD WATER: There's nothing like a dip in nature. You'll deepen relationships with your environment, friends, and yourself, and you can practice without consuming water. Be sure you're getting in a safe, supervised swimming area and that you monitor beach conditions, weather reports, and water quality information. There are some great apps that will tell you the quality of the water (see page 134). I also bring with me a non-contact thermometer so I know what I am getting into.

COLD JOY HOT (OR NOT) TODDY

Not long after we started our cold practice, our son Orren turned twenty-four. We celebrated at Plum Island with a dip, a homemade cake, and warm tea (and an optional shot of bourbon). It's one of my all-time favorite memories. I return to it often in my mind and my mug.

If you've got something to celebrate (you must), there's no better way to warm up than toasting yourself with a toddy.

1 tablespoon lemon juice
1 tablespoon honey (go local!)
½ cup chai tea or hot water
1 ounce bourbon (optional)

Combine the lemon juice and honey in your lucky mug, add the tea or hot water, and stir. Top with the bourbon, if desired.

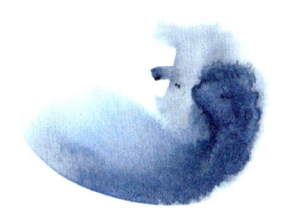

I look back at that first dip (and all my dips since) as an act of curiosity, love, deep listening, trust in my community, and radical self-compassion.

WADING 47

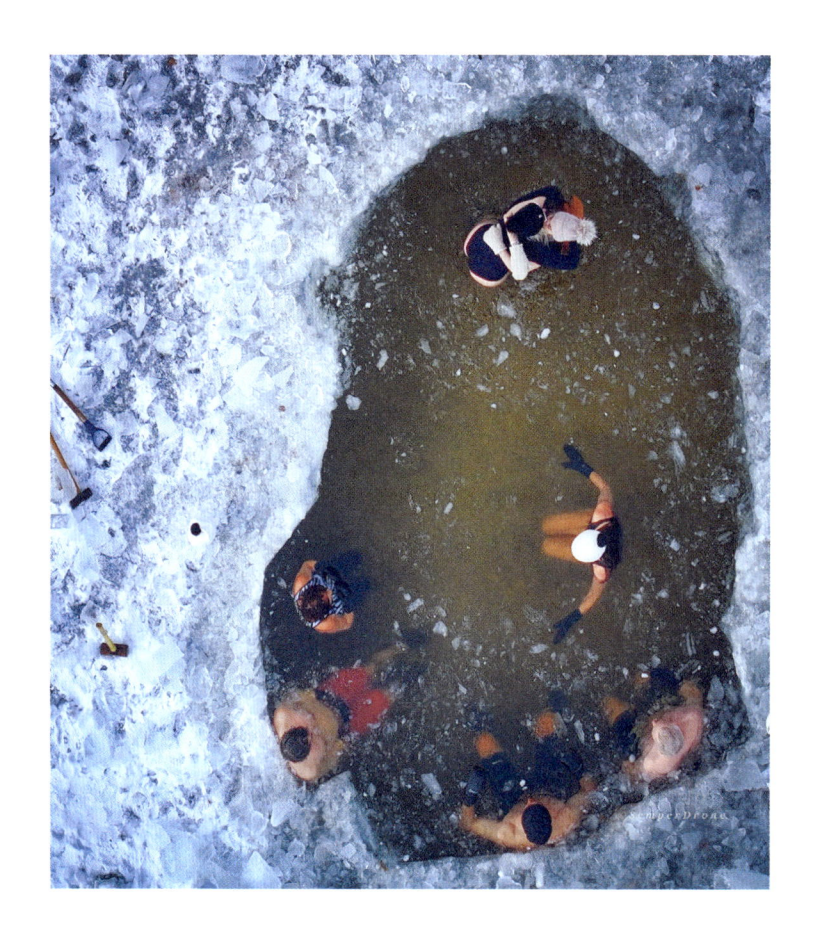

CHAPTER THREE

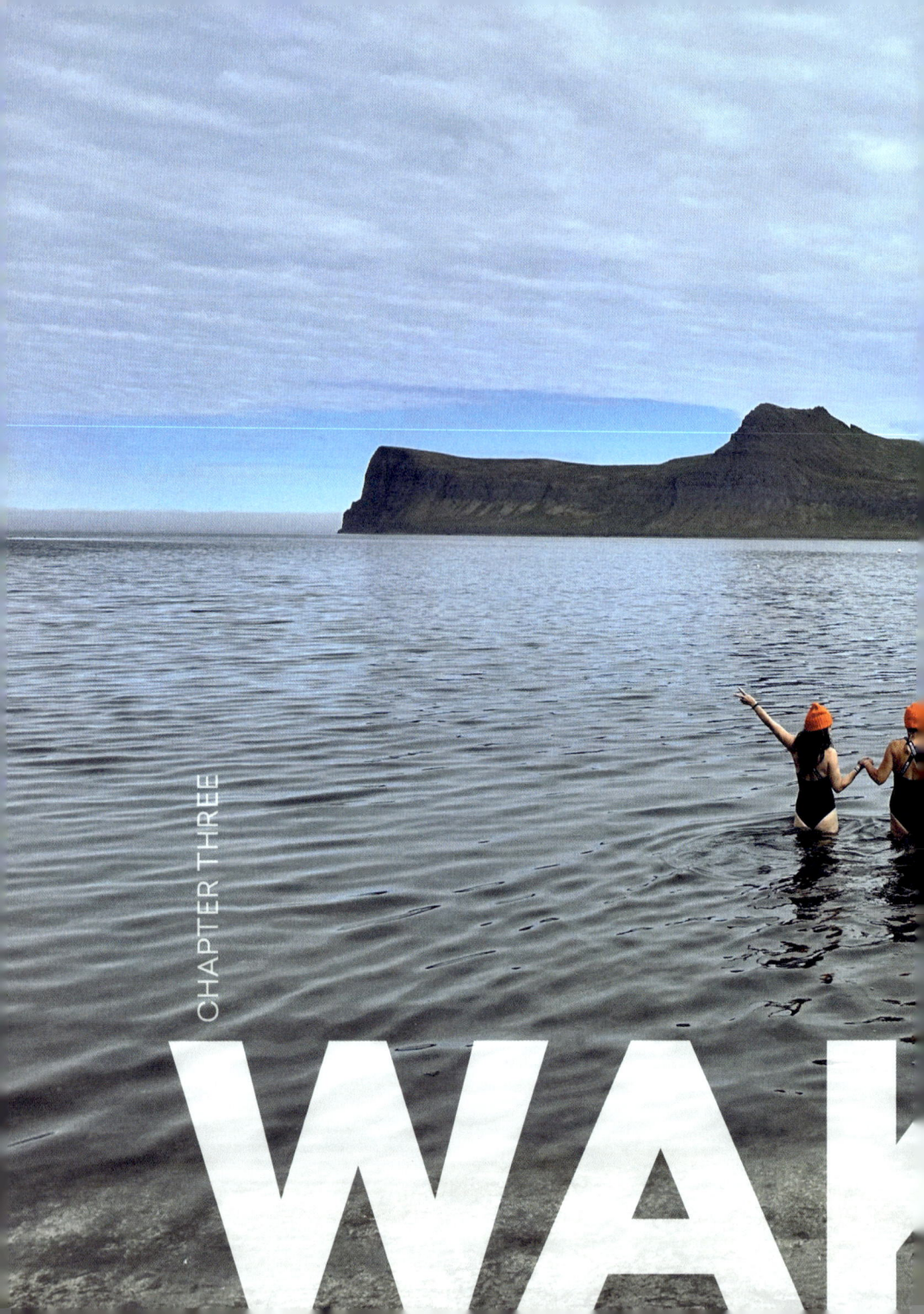

WAK

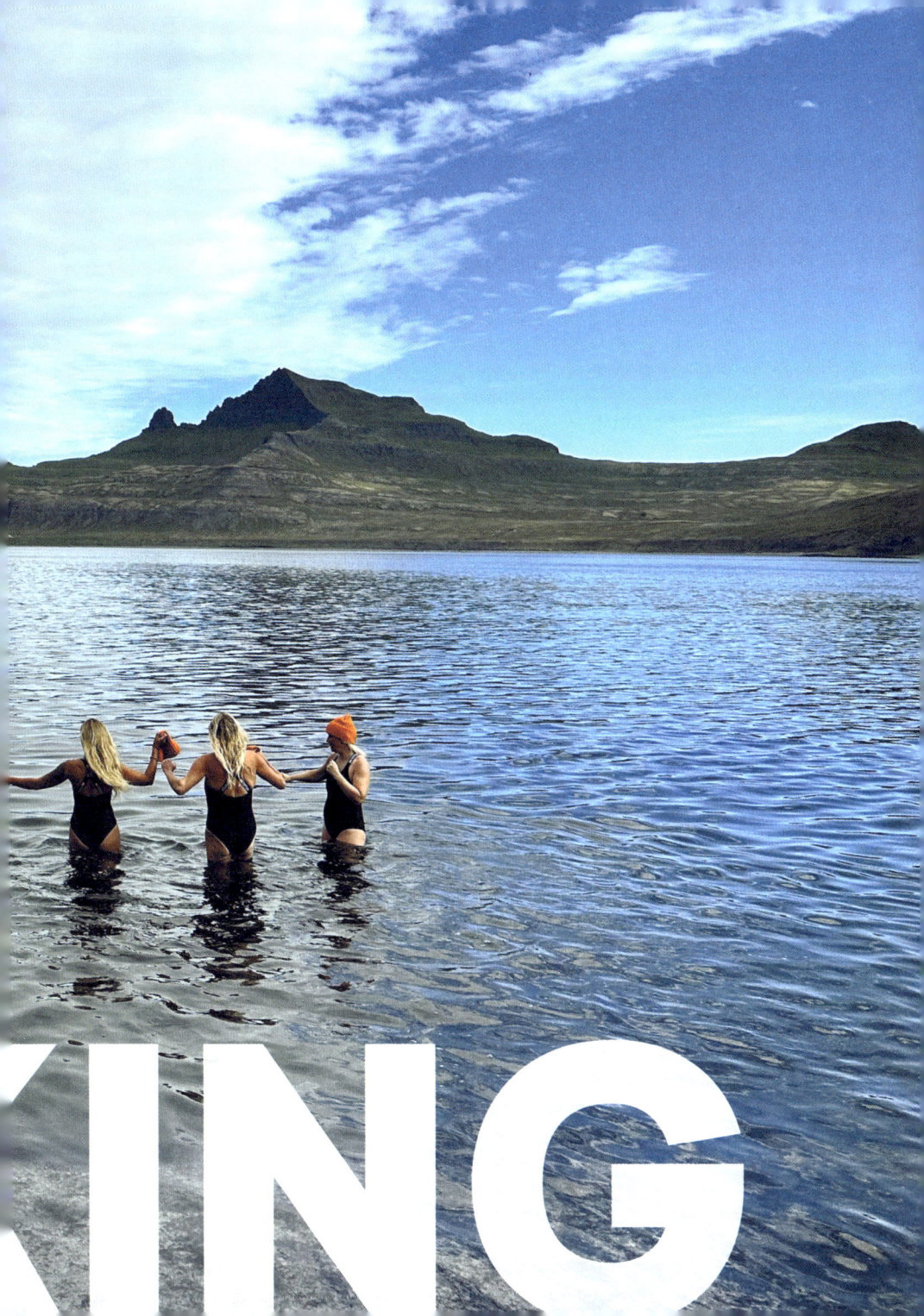

There's a place called Kiruna in the Swedish Lapland, roughly 100 miles above the Arctic Circle. It's filled with birch groves and open tundra. On a March day, the brightness of the shimmering, snow-covered everything is blinding. At night, the place shimmers even more. Look up, and it's as though you can see the entire universe—throbbing flashes of green, thick star cover, purplish smears of galaxy. Look around, and you'll swear the Arctic goes on forever. In the summer, people come to Kiruna to experience the famous midnight sun and fly-fish in the area's thousands of lakes and rivers.

When I visited Kiruna, it was not summer and I was not fishing. The air was a near-constant -7°F (-21°C) and I was mushing dogs fifty kilometers a day, subsisting on freeze-dried rations of bolognese and sleeping in an orange tent so small, you could roll it up and stick it in the pocket of a backpack.

The conditions were extreme, but we had gloves, experience, and smart dogs on our side. Our team was helmed by Tom and Mel, who'd trained for the Iditarod (they loved their dogs fiercely and the dogs were our priority when we arrived at camp). I was wearing all the subzero gear my friends at Fjallraven could throw at me. Once a year, Fjallraven selects twenty individuals from around the world to embark on a sledding trip to show that anyone can be an Arctic explorer. They bring along a few lucky brand ambassadors too. I'd connected with the team through my walking practice and was honored to take part, and terrified too.

My immersion practice (while still emerging) was deeply important to me, and I'd worked hard to change my relationship to the cold. *What if it changed back?*

We started off mid-morning, into a still and peachy sky, each of us with a team of five dogs. Mine were Easy, Bossa, Enzo, Disney, and Nico. Easy was my favorite, and she lived up to her name, grinning through the oppressive, frigid air, yowling for more of it whenever we would break, rolling exuberant and snowy on her back, pink tongue slung out the side of her mouth. She was the embodiment of ease, if not joy, if not ecstasy. I wanted so badly to feel that way, but as the sunscreen froze and the toothpaste froze and I struggled to light the propane stove, the old fears and stories came back. Trauma with a little "t" arrived. I didn't want to be cold anymore. I was scared I wouldn't want to be cold ever again.

After three days of hacking frozen logs of dog food with a hatchet and watching my breath crystalize as it left my mouth, we returned to the lodge on the edge of Lake Väkkärä. The trip was enchanting, breathtaking, and very hard—a grind on the body but a salve on the eyeballs. The experience changed me. I wondered, with an achy heart, how much.

Within an hour of our return, our hosts cut a hole in the ice for us. I'd forgotten we'd asked them to. It was twilight, stupid-mesmerizing, and twinkling. They carved a perfectly square hole in the lake, which was frozen two-feet thick. The edges of the opening were illuminated by reindeer-fat candles that burned like lanterns under translucent shards of ice. They'd left deerskins out to keep our feet warm and slipped a knobbly wooden ladder into the water so that we could enter it gently. Looking at the water, I was emotional. It was something between artwork and home. It was romance and magic and love. It was dogs tossing their heads back and singing to the moon, in what I deeply understood on the top rung of the ladder to be reverence—recognition that cold was a part of them, their identity, their pedigree. It was Easy.

As I slipped into the black viscous water, letting it curl around me like ink, howling in praise on the inside, I recognized that the cold was a part of me too.

LESSON:

Getting Serious About Getting Cold

Cold-water immersion can be a vacation fling or your deepest friendship. It's delicious fun to take part in an annual Polar Plunge with friends or stick your legs into an ice bath after a Sunday long run. For many chill-seekers, that's plenty. But with consistency, care, and community that beautiful feeling of **awakening** we experience when we sink ourselves into the cold and exhale can grow into something more expansive, an **aliveness** we carry not with, but in, us. The cold water can become our solid ground. It has become mine.

I believe any practice should be personal, practical, and powerful. Ultimately, it needs to give more than it takes. When developing your practice, try to think of it as a relationship, not a routine. It may change over time. You may wake up some days liking it more than others. You might take a break and get back together. You might not work out and that's OK! But if you do, celebrate the moments that invite deeper inquiry, take note of any points of tension; experiment and enjoy it.

Your relationship with cold water will look different than mine. And I love that. This is not a rule book, it's a permission slip. Your practice is **yours**—as long as you're happy, healthy, safe, and fulfilled, you're doing it right. Here are some questions that may come up when you're done dipping your toes in and feel ready to go deeper.

HOW OFTEN?
Some cold-water researchers, like Dr. Susanna Søberg, have found that eleven minutes of cold spread out over the course of a week provides ideal benefits. My practice has felt productive with both more and less exposure than that.

When I started to get serious, frequency was much more important than duration to me. I got into the water most days to keep the experience fresh in my mind and familiar to my body. Sometimes, it was a quick in-and-out, other times, I lingered. After a week, the newbie nerves subsided and I genuinely looked forward to my dips. I get in four to five days per week with friends and, for me, that feels like a sweet spot. I have friends who dip twice a week and others who practice daily.

It's a good idea to take inventory of any other practices you maintain. What makes them work? Where do you run into challenges? What do you realistically have time for? Does an economized version of the experience, like a quick cold shower, still provide benefits to you? Do you like taking your time?

I do very well with consistency. I am a systems person. I like being able to depend on my dip. But not everyone is wired like I am. A general rule to follow is that if it starts to feel like work, it's not working. Try something new.

WHEN?
I dip before I chai and I'm convinced a 6:00 A.M. cold dip can make a morning person out of anyone (I have many friends and sons who disagree). There's some early evidence suggesting that an early dip may cause thermogenesis (brown-fat heat production) and spur metabolism along, but I like it because it takes me from weary to wide awake more effectively than black tea and disco music. I love starting my day with friends and a sense of accomplishment and centeredness.

Doing something for myself before the sun has fully risen feels like a bit of a declaration. And I've noticed that if I don't dip early, I'm much more likely to skip it entirely.

If you're not a morning person and have a flexible schedule, a dip can be a wonderful 3:00 P.M. pick-me-up. I have a group of sober friends who swear by cold-water Happy Hour. The only time I don't love a dip is before bed. If I feel too sparkly, I might not sleep. But find what feels right to you—some people love evening in the water.

HOW LONG?

Not too long! Internet iceman culture has made cold exposure into a bit of a contest, but I don't think that's the healthiest or most humble or most honest way to come to the water. As a rule, I don't time my dips. I try to listen to my body and am mindful that I don't stay in longer than I ought to. If I start to feel distracted, unwell, or grumpy, I get out.

Early on, just getting in the water is a great goal. As your practice grows, keep in mind that there's a difference between pushing yourself to the limit and exploring boundaries. Come to the water curious. Don't get burned out on the cold.

HOW COLD?
I generally dip in water colder than 60°F (15°C) and warmer than 35°F (2°C), but it's important to ask your doctor what they feel is safe and to respect that number, even if Joe Internet is plunging for eight minutes at 30°F and ascending to a higher spiritual plane. Do you and only you.

I bring a non-contact thermometer along with me to every cold-water outing to make sure I'm not getting into any water chillier than I can withstand. Through my years of cold dipping, a thermometer helps me understand the energy and dynamics of the water.

IS IT WORKING?
I love to answer this question with a question.

How do you feel?

At the end of each week, I check in with myself and modify my routine if needed. If I feel I'm not getting enough sleep, I might do a shorter dip or switch to cold showers. If I'm feeling bored, I might shake things up with a group dip or head to the beach instead of the tank. If I'm happy and healthy, smiling a little bigger, finding a few extra ounces of empathy and little bits of energy, the practice is working perfectly **for me**.

THE LAST DROP

You can deepen your practice by mushing dogs across the Arctic Circle (highly recommended) or you can skip the orange tent and frozen propane-stove tea and simply work to approach the water each day with curiosity and commitment. It *will* be cold, but what else could it be? Enlivening? Joyful? Challenging? Fun? Developing a relationship with the cold water—not just a routine— has kept me engaged, awakened, always looking forward to the next dip.

KALLBADHUS CULTURE

After three days of dog sledding in the Arctic, we felt a little silly asking our hosts at Lake Väkkärä if we could wait on the mulled wine and go jump in the lake, but they didn't bat an eye. Cold-bathing culture has been alive and well in Sweden—and in many other Nordic countries—since the nineteenth century, if not earlier.

Along the coast and in many of the nation's lakes and rivers, you can find a kallbadhus, or cold-swimming club, and a community that loves it.

KALLBADHUS culture is:

CONTRAST-BASED: Many bathers follow their cold dip with a sauna (or vice versa!), enjoying the benefits of both practices.

OUTDOORS: Wild water is where my heart is. Most bathhouses make use of the country's exquisite natural water, and with 97,500 lakes and 2,000 miles of coastline, there's plenty to choose from.

KALLBADHUS CULTURE cont'd

SOCIAL: Cold bathing is seen as much more than a wellness practice, it's a way to unwind with friends, strengthen community, and meet people. Many bathhouses have a restaurant on premise so bathers can share a meal or a drink after their dip. *Skål!*

(OFTEN) CLOTHING OPTIONAL: I know which option I'd choose.

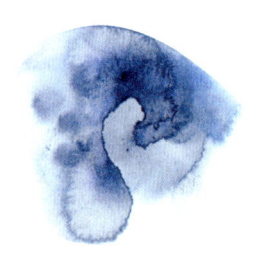

Your practice is yours—
as long as you're happy,
healthy, safe, and fulfilled,
you're doing it right.

WIT

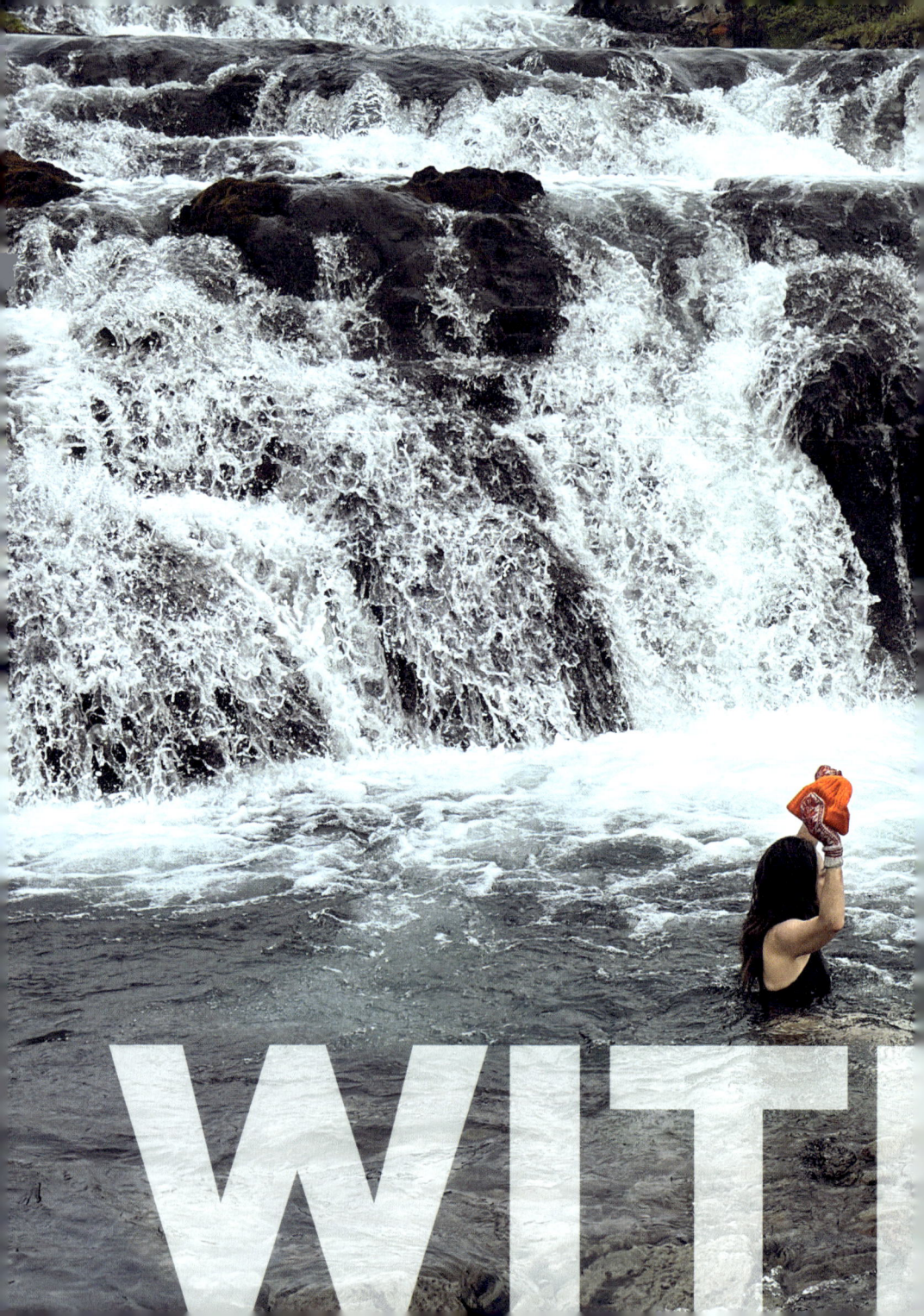

CHAPTER FOUR

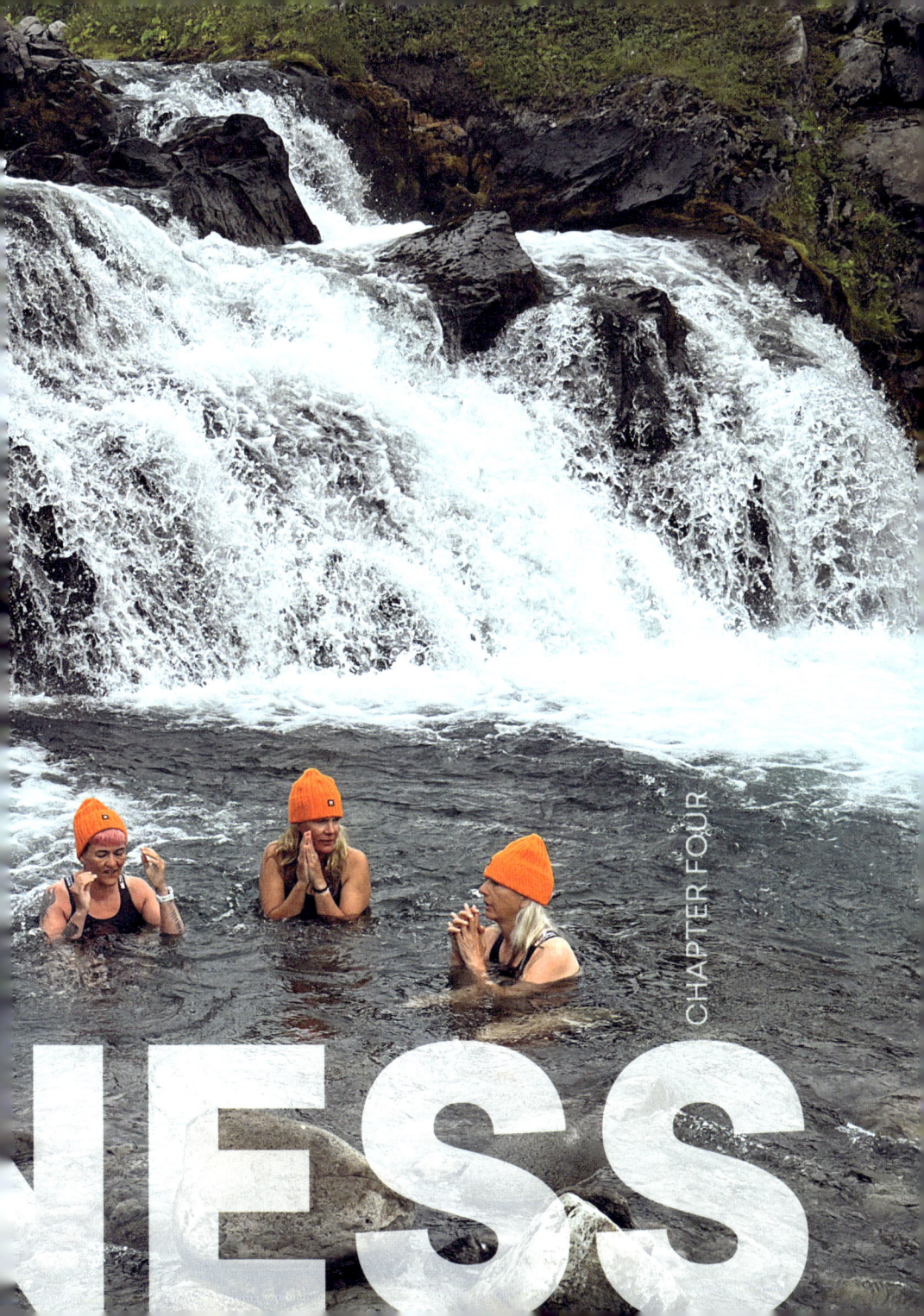

NESS

From a certain vantage, the White Mountains in New Hampshire look like a field of perfect women resting on their sides—luxuriating, Rubenesque, and kissed by the light. Some have their giant, granite heads propped up on fists of rock and others seem as though they're laughing, chins tilted back, the sharpness of their noses and teeth piercing the blue winter sky. One bluff leans into another to whisper her most delicious secret. The other bats her cedar lashes, weeping in joyful rivers down the ruggedness of her cheeks and chest, all the way out to the ocean. The secret between them, I've always guessed, is "I love you." And isn't that the most delicious secret of all?

I spent the first days of December 2023 tucked into the contours of this magical Wabanaki land, dancing down the trail with six mermaids, searching for a perfect pool of water. Contrary to popular belief, mermaids make excellent hikers.

Mermaids are thoughtful, silly, brilliant, gentle, and deep. They are ding-dongs, geniuses, and wild, slightly feral children. They are some of my very best friends on earth. "Mermaid" is the term many of us use to describe the members of our cold-dipping communities. And yes, men can be mermaids too. Dipping together is an intimate act. It's a vulnerable and radical promise to let others in, all the way. Getting in the water in community is like singing in a choir, lifting the voices around you, and allowing yourself to be lifted. I am much better at one of those things than the other.

The air temperature at the trailhead was in the low-forties, and as we dipped our fingers in the streams and springs we passed, we could guess the water was about the same. Ari, a very wise mermaid and an experienced outdoorsman, led us down the trail in our crampons and swimsuits. It was exciting and joyful, and we giggled and danced over ice-smothered rocks and new mosses, celebrating something that hadn't happened yet.

"Libby, look!" Ari said.

She pointed her mitten toward a dark corner of the stream where the current was calm. A small, white waterfall spilled gently down a limestone stairway and made its landing, eddying around a few smooth stones. We stripped down to our suits, checked the water temperature, and, one by one, slipped into a gentle flow, breathing the pine sap, mud, and minerally granite deep in our lungs. I was among the last to get in.

I'm a tough cookie. And back then, in the season of fortification that often follows a season of loss, I was defiantly tough, always wearing invisible armor under my fuzzy sweater. I took pride in being able to care for myself and my people. I loved how much I didn't need and didn't take. Or wouldn't admit to needing anyway. I took off my boots, my snow pants, and my big jacket. I took off my fuzzy sweater. I turned around and saw six hands outstretched toward me, but the approach looked smooth, so I didn't grab ahold.

I slipped into the water. It was colder than I had expected. It took my breath away and something like panic happened. I hadn't reacted to the cold this way in a long time. It was more of a dull ache than a homecoming. As I lowered all the way in, I had to shut my eyes. I reached back for the hands that were so generously reaching for me and heard, "you got this" and "breathe" and "I love you, Lib." I kept my eyes closed for a long time. When I opened them, I saw love—Sarah, who taught me to laugh down to my toes. Suze, who taught me to cry big tears in the company of others. Ari and Kimmie, who were still holding my hands. I had never felt so desperately not alone. We can find ourselves in the water. And we can find each other too.

We sang and danced and cheered, and afterward we ate beautiful homemade chocolate-chip cookies and drank hot tea on the soft banks of the stream. That day, the water showed me parts of myself I never knew existed— tenderness, fear, need. The mermaids and the water taught me to trust and love them.

MERMAID
MAGIC

Stepping into this practice with others is entering into an ecosystem of generosity, where care, skill, earth wisdom, and affection are communal resources, often humbling in their abundance. There's a culture of familial love, a sense of being watched over and believed in, cherished, even. I know there will be an extra sweater if I need it. I know that if my expression changes, someone will ask if I'm OK. If I need encouragement, it will be there, likely before I can ask for it.

The social culture of cold exposure goes back (at least!) to the Roman baths, where citizens of all social standings and walks of life were welcome to relax together. In these spaces, many of the lines that defined ancient society were obscured: the rich bathed with the poor, the young with the old. This spirit endures and continues to expand. I've met so many people in the water that I never would have met otherwise. I have friends who teach preschool and friends who teach yoga, comedian friends and kayaker friends, friends in broken places and friends in whole ones. I dip with tree huggers and ex-cons. We come from all different faiths, races, and places, and the water has room for all of us. It is in all of us. We have so much to learn from one another. The water is a brilliant teacher that attracts brilliant teachers.

There are plenty of practical reasons to get in the water together too. Cold-water communities can help us stay accountable and add an extra layer of safety to the experience. In an emerging practice, they offer mentorship and motivation; in an established one, they keep things from getting stale, bringing variety to the practice as well as exposure to new techniques, new locations, and new mindsets. They're also a heck of a lot of fun. And we should always come to water with fun, shouldn't we?

Mermaid communities dip to disco music and in Santa hats. They howl at the full moon. They celebrate birthdays on the beach with cake and sparklers, then get in the water, form a circle, and sing to the birthday mermaid in the middle. On Sundays we read Mary Oliver's *Why I Wake Early* aloud and, I swear, it's the best kind of church I've ever been to. Many people like the responsibility and expectation that come with being a "member," but for me, it's the opposite. Being in the water together is like coming home from school. I show up as I am. The time for performance has passed. Would I like a hug? Absolutely.

And then there's the greatest show on earth: Perhaps the deepest value in community practice lies in the earnest, near-cosmic connection born when we welcome each other into the water, witnessing the vulnerability and victory held in that moment of entry, of arrival. We learn to give and receive, to hold space and to occupy it. We get to watch one another grow, and there is nothing more beautiful.

LESSON:

How to Be a Mermaid

My friends at Ebb & Flow (@ebb.and.flow.collective and @ebb.and.flow.collective.sf) are expert cold-water community makers. They've taken a group of wild, slightly feral women in bathing suits and neoprene booties and made us into a proper family. They've built a culture that's kind, committed, and quirky, but behind all the disco dips and cake by the ocean, there's some serious decorum too. These are the rules we (live and) dip by:

DON'T COMPARE: Every body is different and so is every practice. Some days, you may look around and be tempted to stay in longer than you should. You might feel badly about your level of tolerance. You might even feel bashful about the perfectly magical way your bathing suit clings to your body. Instead, focus on what you all have in common—the water, care of the community, commitment to ourselves and to this glorious place.

SHARE! I keep a stash of woolies and warmies in the back of my car just in case anyone needs an extra layer to keep warm after their dip. I also like to bring along an extra thermos of tea on an especially cold day. It's an easy way to look out for your people and make somebody's day. I've never brought the extra thermos home full.

DON'T INSTRUCT: What works for you, may not work for your fellow mermaid. Some dippers like to keep their eyes wide open, others squeeze them shut. Some like to swim, others stay still. Some are conversationalists, others are quiet as mice. If someone asks for guidance, feel free to contribute, but don't try to direct somebody else's experience. Only intervene if you see someone endangering themselves or others.

ENCOURAGE! Getting in the water is an act of bravery every single time. Show your mermaids—new and old—some great, big love. Tell them how amazing they are. Tell them how happy you are that they came. Tell them how much they inspire you. Hold their hand if they need a little support. Dearest mermaid Sarah started a practice of hugging all the time. Every dip. We all need hugs.

DON'T BE SHY: Introduce yourself. Let your fellow dippers know your name, your experience level, and what brought you to the water. Get to know those around you. Intros might seem unnecessary, but they're an important first step in staying safe. If something should happen, it's crucial that someone else knows who you are. Plus, it's harder to cheer you on without a name.

SHAKE IT! Be your weird, true, authentic self. Wear the polka-dot bikini. Bring your pom-pom beanie. Say "I love you" out loud. The water loves you. We love you too.

THE LAST DROP

My cold-water community has brought more warmth to my life than I ever could have expected, along with a rich knowledge, a sense of confidence in myself and my practice, and quite a few new dance moves. I've become more expressive. I've learned to lift others and, crucially, to let others lift me. I don't just plan on asking for help. I practice. The cold water is filled with tough cookies, but all it takes is a little mermaid magic to get to the tender middle. Everyone knows that's the best part.

I DIP, YOU DIP, WE DIP

The fastest way to get a group of people in ski jackets excited about getting in the water is the perfect playlist. And yes, it's water-themed.

- "Da' Dip" by Freak Nasty
- "Water" by Tyla
- "Ocean Eyes" by Billie Eilish
- "Cry Me a River" by Justin Timberlake
- "Cold as Ice" by Foreigner
- "Cake by the Ocean" by DNCE
- "Drink Water" by Jon Batiste
- "Cold hard B****" by Jet
- "Water" by Salatiel, Pharrell Williams, Beyoncé
- "Ocean" by Martin Garrix feat. Khalid
- "Take Me to the River" by Al Green
- "Moon River" by Frank Ocean
- "Down By the Water" by The Decemberists
- "If I Had a Boat" by Lyle Lovett
- "River" by Leon Bridges
- "Cold Water" by Damien Rice
- "The Sea and the Rhythm" by Iron & Wine
- "Hold Back the River" by James Bay

WITCHY SH*T

Women and water have a wild and supernatural history. From sirens and Celtic river goddesses to Mami Wata (Mother Water) and the Lady of the Lake, feminine spirits flow through folklore in wells, rivers, lakes, and oceans, often symbolic of fertility, healing, power, and wisdom.

But there are a few chapters in our history that are less fantastical.

In seventeenth-century Europe and parts of America, "swimming a witch" was a tactic used to prove whether an individual was involved with black magic or consorting with the devil. First outlawed in the Middle Ages, trial by water, or judicium aquae frigidae ("ordeal of the cold water"), was outlawed, but it reemerged under James I, who praised the practice in his wildly paranoid, witch-hunting how-to Daemonologie, which gets a baffling 3.59 rating on Goodreads.

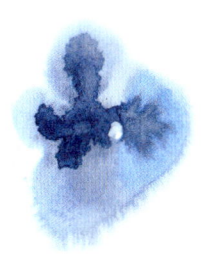

WITCHY SH*T cont'd

Magistrates would tie up the "afflicted" and throw her in the open water. If she sank, it was proof of her innocence. If she floated, she was deemed guilty and often hanged.

Don't worry, James I died of dysentery. And we've since taken back our witchiness, our water, and our power. One-hundred percent recommend a witchy dip with your mermaids!

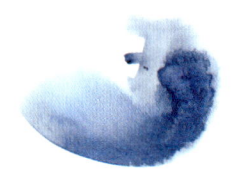

Be your weird, true, authentic self. Wear the polka-dot bikini. Bring your pom-pom beanie. Say "I love you" out loud. The water loves you. We love you too.

CHAPTER FIVE

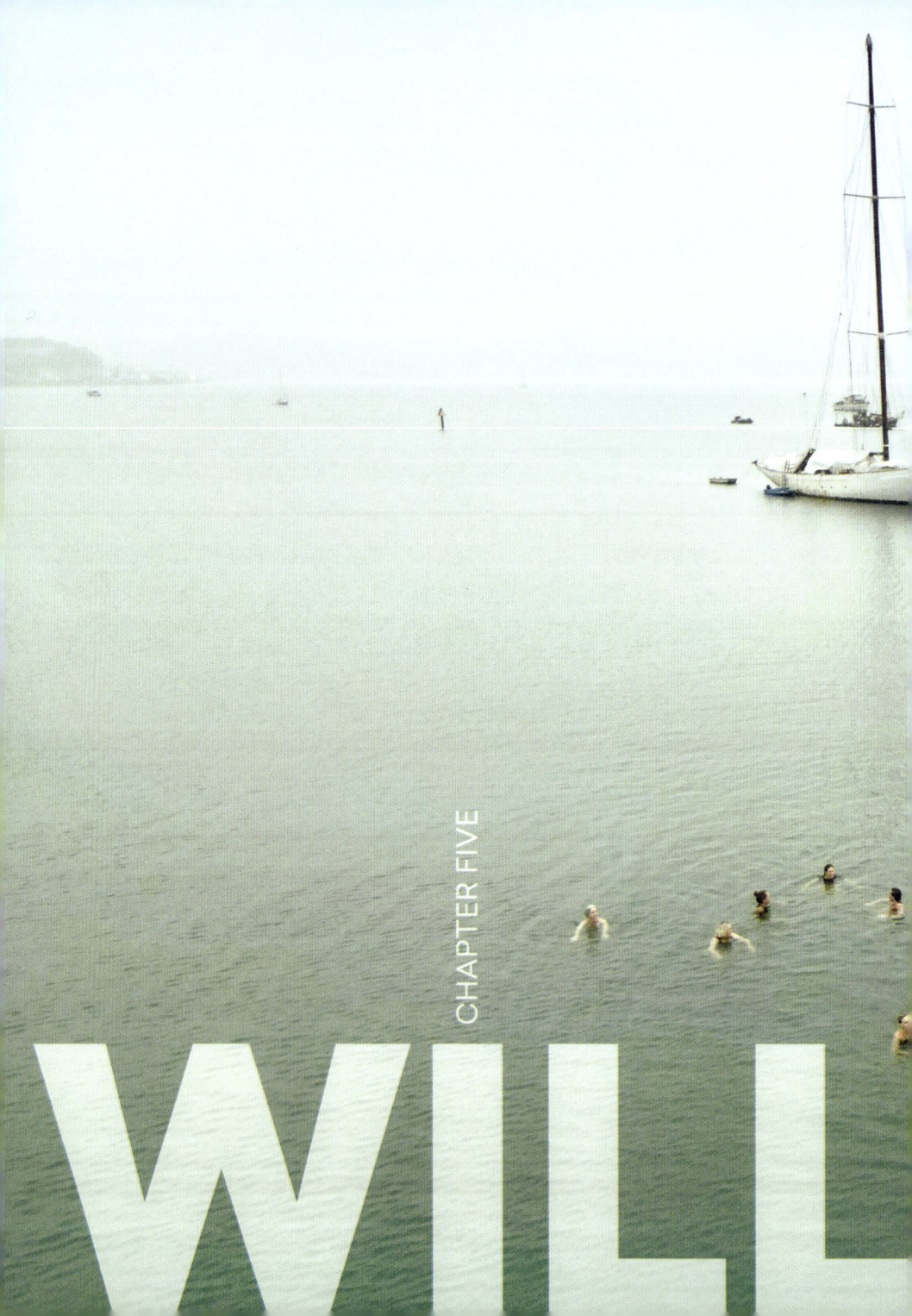

WILL

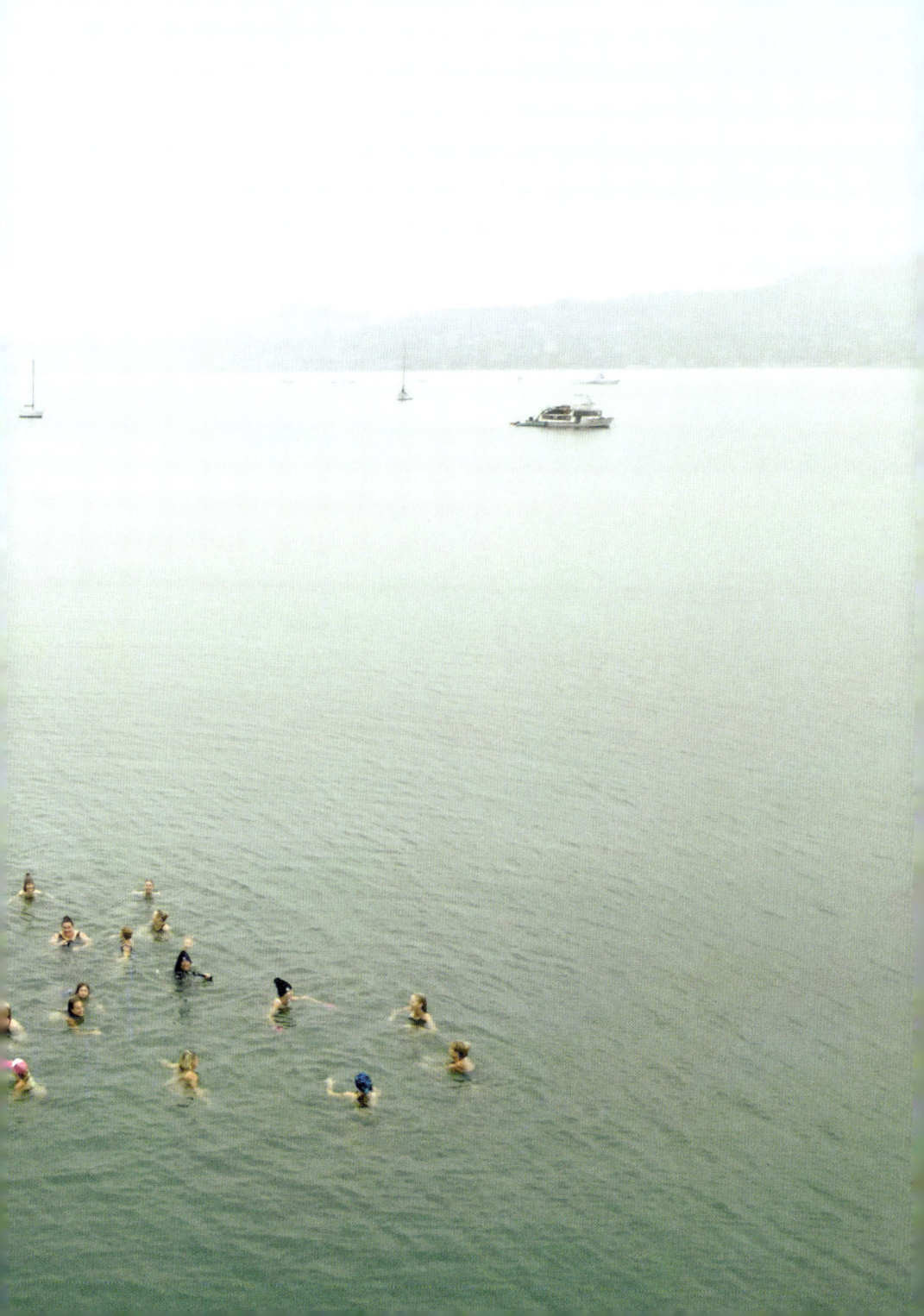

April has always been kind, except for once, when she was a bully. The weather in Newburyport, Massachusetts, was particularly gray that month, with low, goading clouds and shrill winds packed with peppery drops of ice and snow and sand. None of the flowers opened, but all the winter birds had gone. For weeks, we were lost in time, stuck in the hinterland between winter and spring, neither season waving her hands on the horizon. The mermaids, understandably, were frustrated.

There was rain. So much rain, and every single kind of rain you could think of. Normally, wetness isn't the sort of thing to derail watery people, but for pioneering communities like Lowell, Massachusetts, and Manchester, New Hampshire, who live on the Merrimack River, downstream from the fount of the American Industrial Revolution, big rain means poor water quality. The sewer systems are old. During heavy precipitation and snow melts, the storm and wastewater levels exceed the capacity of sewage and treatment networks, so the excess dumps out into the river. Swimming isn't safe. The local water officials call it a combined sewer overflow, but I have a different term for it that I'll share with you one day over tea.

More persistent than wise, we planned each day to meet at our spot, a small crook in the river lined with skinny trees and smooth pebbles. The water there is calm enough for dipping but still dynamic and tidal. In the early morning, if you concentrate hard enough, you can feel the pull of the moon around your ankles. Many years into the practice, I still get butterflies when I drive up to this beach and shut down the engine. After about a week of planning and canceling and waiting for conditions to improve, with nothing but rain before and behind us in the forecast, Sarah, a tenured mermaid, made the call via text message.

"I think we have to go solo. Tank time."

At the time, community and cold exposure were synonymous to me. The people were an integral part of the practice. There were hands to hold, eyes to lock onto during the first big ache, peals of laughter that made everything sparkle brighter. The water and people in it were woven together so tightly in my heart, it felt impossible to unravel one from the other. But completely against my will and because April made me, I was going to have to practice my cold exposure alone.

Dutifully but with little enthusiasm, I accepted a 2×2×4 stock tank from the generous Mary-Jo, who decided she wasn't going to use it. I stuck the tub in my backyard and filled it up with the garden hose under a snowy sky and the curious (likely concerned) gaze of my neighbor Bill. When I was done, I stood back and took it in. It was unfriendly, still, and steel. Nothing had ever looked less like a river. Naturally, the night before the maiden voyage, there was a freeze.

At 5:00 A.M., in my swimsuit and headlamp, I grabbed Bill's sledgehammer and began hacking away at the thick skin of ice that had formed on the surface of the tub. It was a thunderous process, like ringing a gong. I could hardly see through the steam from my nose and skin, and by the time I managed to carve a Libby-sized hole into the ice, I was sweaty and shivering. It felt like work. It *was* work.

I laid out my bathmat, kicked my boots off into the snow, and took it all in—dead water next to a dead garden; dim, starless sky; metal bucket full of loneliness; and no one waiting for me in the water.

With wooly mittened hands, I grabbed the corners of the tank and submerged quickly up to my neck. I don't recommend getting in this way to anyone, at any point in your practice. There was nothing gentle or kind about my motions. I used my body like a knife. Getting into the water *hurt*. I was *hurting*.

During the first few seconds, I would have given anything for anyone, even Bill, to save me, but whatever it was I needed, I was going to have to find it myself. I did my best to picture a soothing mother figure or a spirit or a friend, but improbably the most comforting image I could find was a no-nonsense version of myself, in a sturdy blue sweater and fabulously big glasses.

Get to calm, Lib. You're almost there. Breathe, her/my voice said, *you're doing it.*

Then I spoke the words out loud: "You are safe. You. Are. Safe. Exhale. Get to calm."

I kept my eyes shut and looked further inward to my own steadying gaze, the partner within myself. We breathed rhythmically, together. We held each other. We got to calm, and calm was a mountain that day. These seconds were long and worrying, but as the time passed, so did the fear, the longing, the hurting.

We did it, or I did.

By the time I opened my eyes, there was enough light in the sky that I could make out a stark but beautiful shadow of my reflection. She had been waiting in the water all along. "I love you."

LESSON:

Going Solo (in a Tank/Tub)

A solo dip in a galvanized tank feels very different than a wild, communal one. The energy is more intense. I wouldn't call it excitement, but acute focus. Practicing alone is harder (for me). It requires total presence and invites deeper inquiry. There's no one there to drown out the voice reminding you that you don't like the cold or questioning if you're brave enough. You're confronted with your own noise and challenged to find your own quiet. This is where I truly learned to "get to calm."

Many people without access to wild water or cold-water communities begin their dipping journey alone. If this had been the case for me, I'm sure I'd still be on the other side of the starting line. If this is the case for you, you are a rockstar-superhero-spacewoman. You **can** do it and it **will** be incredible. There's no place to hide, no hand to hold, so many ways out, and no way in but **your** way. I know plenty of dippers who integrate solo time into their practice and come to prefer it for the mental challenge and meditative work they do in the tank. I'm not quite there yet, but it's growing on me.

While you may love it (or not) for a different set of reasons than I do, these are some perks of a solo practice:

NO DISTRACTIONS: Without giggles and sparklers and witch hats and ABBA, I see everything, and I feel everything—good and bad. Mine is the only voice in the room. I can truly listen to what my mind and body have to say and work to become a better listener.

NO DRAMA: Truthfully, there is never any real drama with mermaids, but with a solo dip, you don't even have to worry about logistics! There's no need to pick up doughnuts (but you should) or sit in traffic because your water tank is right there. You're always on time. You get to pick the music. Want to practice breathwork in the tank? Sing? Splash? Have at it!

BIG DISCIPLINE: Commitment is one of the three pillars of Iceman Wim Hof's cold-immersion method, and while my practice is quite different from his, I acknowledge that commitment is breathtakingly hard. Dipping alone has meant learning to make and keep promises to myself, without relying on anyone else to hold me accountable. It has also meant I need to be intentional in caring for myself. Before every dip, I have to ask an important question: **Lib, what do you need?** On a basic level, I need to be sure my towel is easily accessible, since there won't be anyone there to pass it my way, and I need to be sure I'm dipping safely, with a cell phone and a buddy nearby. I also need my tea.

BIG-DIP ENERGY: I am proud of my solo practice, and every time I climb Calm Mountain, I feel a massive sense of accomplishment, a supercharged confidence I carry with me through the rest of the day. Maybe it's the endorphins, maybe it's the tea, but when I dip alone, I swear there's something special in the water. Maybe it's me?

LESSON:

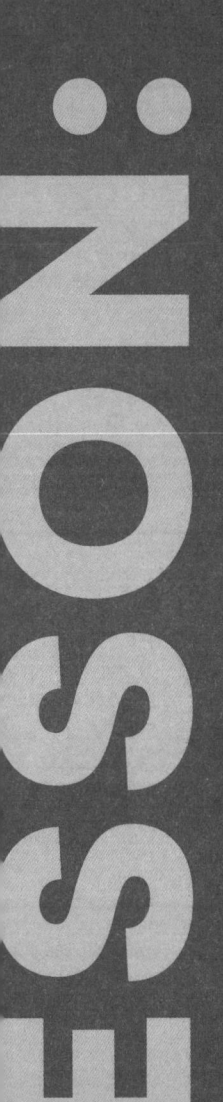

Fresh Air

Breathwork is the best work. It's been instrumental in helping me connect with my body and stay strong and focused in the water. For me, a breathing pattern is a place to return when things veer off course in the tank (they will! It's OK!). You might get anxious. You might hear a cool owl or have a negative thought. You might just be feeling a little scattered. Breathwork isn't for everyone and it isn't something you need to integrate into your practice if it doesn't appeal to you, but it's been an excellent tool to keep me where I need to be—right here, right now.

Here are a few of my favorite techniques:

BOX BREATHING: Breathe in to a count of four. Hold your breath to a count of four. Exhale to a count of four. Hold for four. You can picture a box (or a present) while doing this. This technique may be hard to sustain in the water, but it's a great way to gear up for a dip and a grounding pattern to repeat if you're struggling in the water.

CANDLE BREATHING: A dear little friend brought this pattern home from kindergarten after a day of big feelings. Take a deep breath in through the nose for a count of four, then blow out for even longer (ideally, to a count of eight) through pursed lips. Aim for the candle on your cake. Can you see it? Everything, including visualization, is better with cake.

EXTENDED EXHALE: When you hit the water, especially if you're new to the practice, your body might panic. When this happens to me and counting isn't possible, I come back to my exhales. I exhale powerfully, longer than my inhale, and I do it audibly, like Old Man Winter.

DIAPHRAGMATIC BREATHING: Sometimes called "belly breathing," diaphragmatic breathing concentrates on using the domed shaped muscle at the bottom of your lungs to drive the breathing motion. Picture filling your belly, not your chest. Breathe in and let your belly move out; breathe out and let your belly soften inward. Some people keep a hand on their chest and belly while doing this breath, but I find it difficult in the water.

THE LAST DROP

I'm not always good at keeping promises to myself. I feel this tendency loud and clear in my solo practice, especially on an inky, dark-blue winter morning when I'm tucked in bed and the tank is waiting for me outside, frozen thick. But I get up, dust off my sleepies, quiet my snarlies, and go outside. I grab Bill's sledgehammer (he doesn't bother to put it in his shed anymore) and carve a space for myself in the ice. That's really what the solo practice is all about, making space for *you*.

LESSON: Get to Calm

Calm is peace, calm is courage, calm is the top of the mountain. Come with me, I'll hold your hand.

QUIET BREATH: Pick a breathing pattern that feels comfortable and centering. I like to practice a few cycles before I get in and try to continue through the first uncomfortable moments of cold.

QUIET BRAIN: Choose an image that feels peaceful, or that might correspond to your breathing pattern. I know a lot of dippers who like to imagine a campfire flickering. I also know a few mermaids who picture of all things, the water.

QUIET BODY: Try to get still. It's easy to want to wiggle your way to warm, but there is so much joy in just letting the water hold you. Resist the urge to grip the edges of the tub/tank or curl your toes. Just be.

QUIET HEART: It's likely that (1) you came to the water with something on your heart (a thought, a feeling, a wish, a hope), or (2) you found something the second you got in. Release it. Even if it's just for now. Release might look like laughter or tears or funny animal sounds. It might be a primal scream. Let it all out.

Welcome to Calm. You'll love it here.

By the time I opened my eyes, there was enough light in the sky that I could make out a stark but beautiful shadow of my reflection. She had been waiting in the water all along. "I love you."

CHAPTER SIX

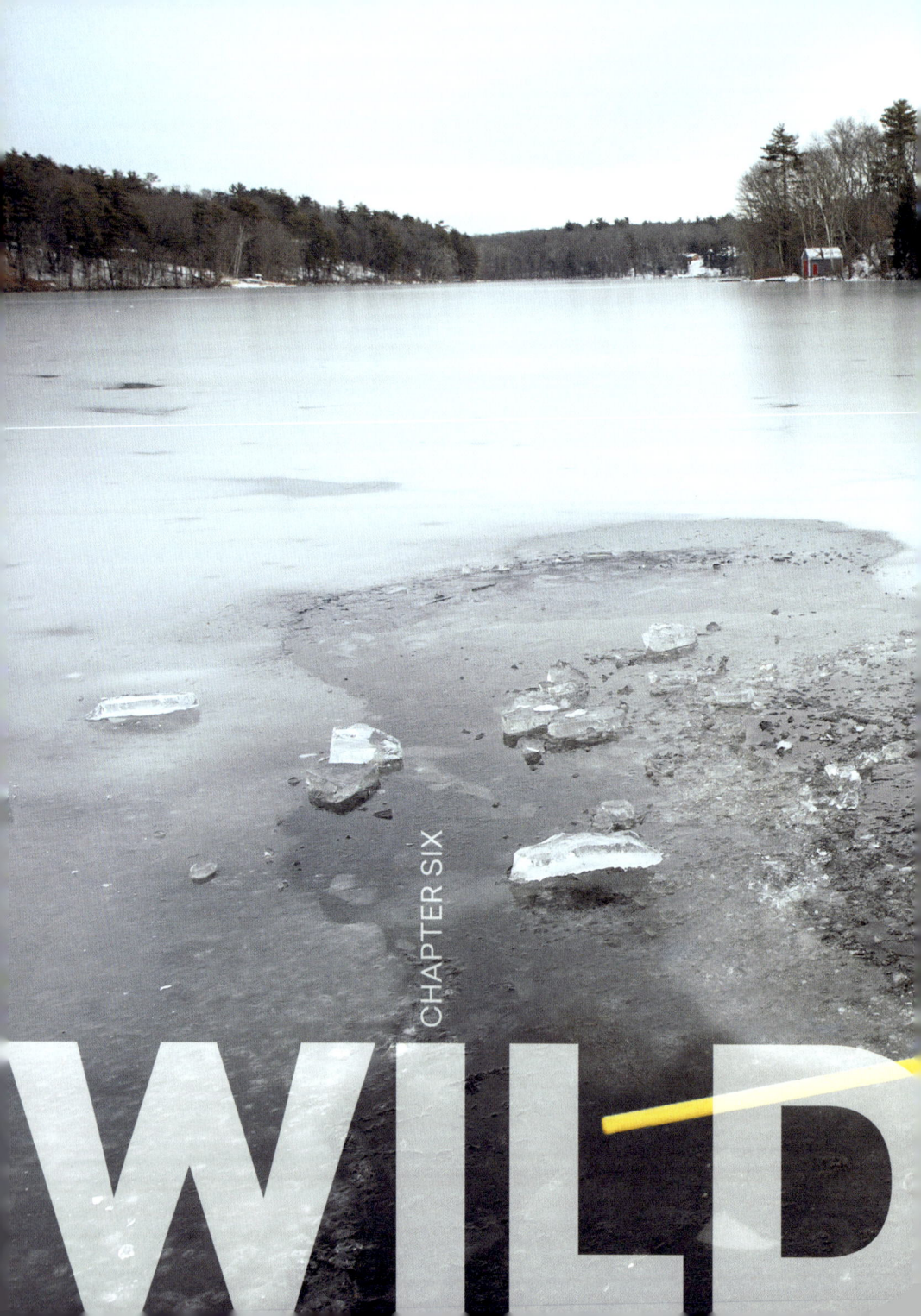

WILD

NESS

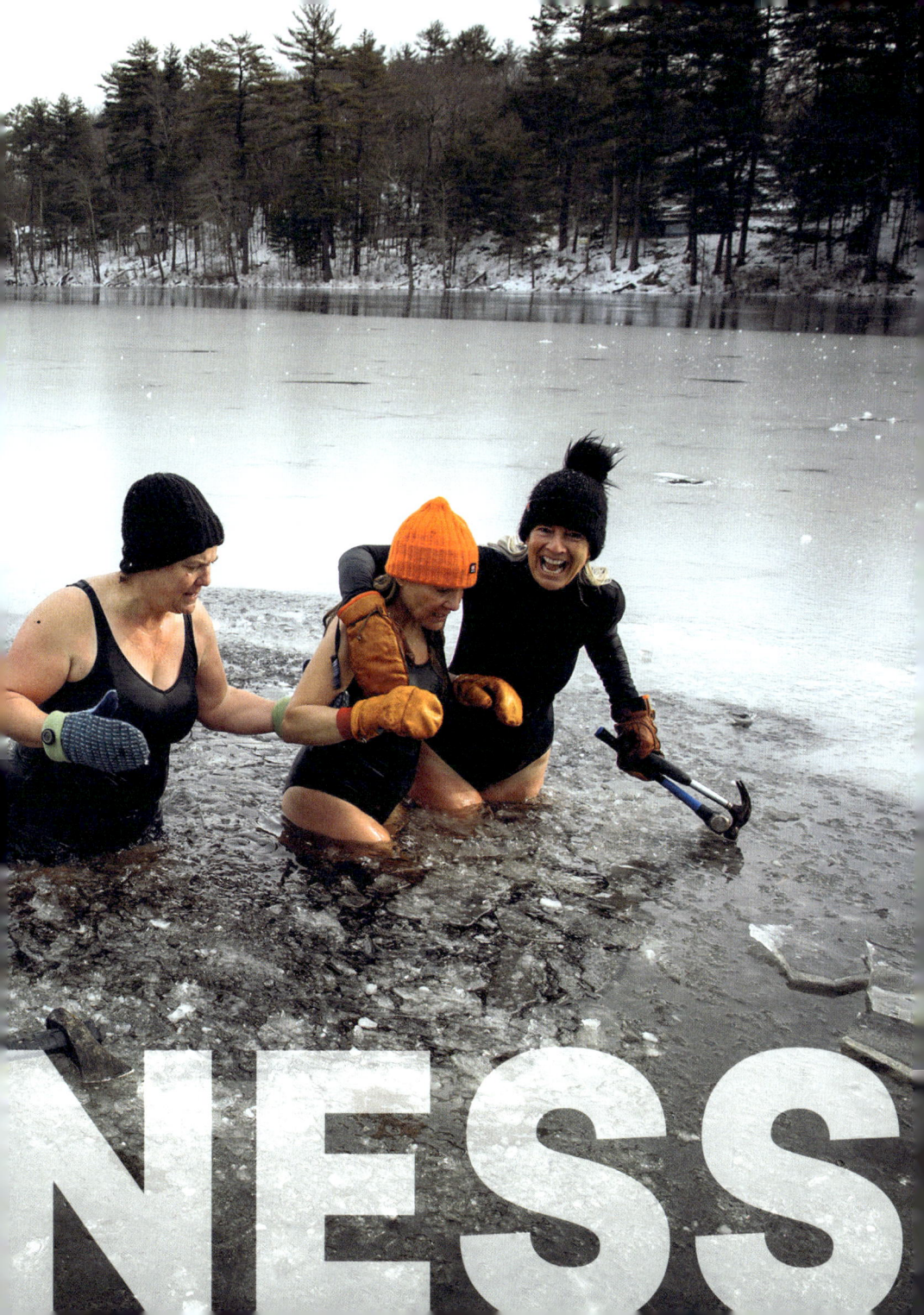

Every time I dip in Sausalito, California, I think to myself, *There's a lot of wild in this water.*

It smells wild, the sulphury brine a mix of wet sand, new seaweed, big city, and eucalyptus.

It feels wild, rushing toward me unafraid, inviting me in twinkling overtures farther from shore. There is a sense that anything could change at any time. And it *could* change, because this water, like me, is ever-changing and alive. It seems to want and wonder and reach, just as I do.

Our little beach isn't remote or striking to look at. There's a parking lot, a place to recycle your plastic, and a sign with written rules about dogs and swimming after dusk. The beach isn't punctuated by jagged cliffs or rimmed with sharp edges the way the "California Coast" lives in our minds. There's a marina to the right filled with bobbing houseboats and teeny skiffs. Kayakers launch each morning from the silver-gold sand, and toddlers come by after breakfast to excavate imaginary treasures and bottle caps with their pink plastic shovels. The squads of brown pelicans perched on the docks are so used to and fond of humans, they seem disappointed if you don't stop to take their photo. I wave to them most mornings as they fly overhead in a shared "good morning."

But we come to the shore, even in our humble, weekday ways, to stand on the edge of something beautiful, to dip our toes in the otherworld. The beach is wild and the woman with her new puppy is wild—so are the calm grey pelicans and the harbormaster. I'm wild too, up to my hips in the black water, standing under the first pink smudge of daylight and the fading shadow of the big sexy moon.

One foggy morning in September, I arrived early at the water's edge for a dip with friends. I walked onto the beach by myself and took the morning in like breath, listening to boats bump up against their slips, to the fluttering of the flags on their masts. I checked the water temperature. It was 53 degrees. San Francisco Bay stays on the warm side of cold, usually in the mid-fifties year-round. The other mermaids emerged from the parking lot and we hugged hello. A lone kayaker slipped into the water and disappeared into the low morning fog; a man drinking coffee sat on a bench, watching the water. We began to walk into the bay, in clusters of two or three. I went on my own just behind Hilah and Allison and Lucie. I felt something, a presence with me.

We always have more company than we think we do in the water. At any given time, we're swimming alongside a hundred hidden creatures—small silverfish, floating bugs, and snails in turret-shaped shells that tuck away when they hear us coming. Thinking about that gives me butterflies, though I know it gives some people the scaries. That day, most of the mermaids stayed close to shore, but I went a little farther out. I'd memorized the contours of the seafloor at this point, I knew its falls and rises, where it got woolly with weeds. When the water crested my shoulders, the presence felt stronger. I noticed a seal swimming toward me, spinning her long, freckled body through the bay, black marble eyes fixed on mine. It was like we'd agreed to meet right there. She'd been looking forward to it all week.

Harbor seals love this sweet beach. We see them weekly and like to wave to them as they go by, gigantic but moving with shocking grace through the bay. They usually give us a wide berth and we do the same. As a rule, we never approach wildlife and tread lightly wherever we are, understanding that every time we step into the water, we're entering someone's home. I have frequent creature encounters during my walking practice, but it's very different in the ocean. On land, there's a sameness to us. The path, the road, and the forest are common spaces, and there's rarely a gray squirrel excited or surprised to see me. In the water, I'm an interloper, but that morning, for some reason, I felt so much like I'd been invited.

"Sunny" the seal was still moving toward me. Surer of my breath than seal body language, I became still and waited, signaling to my friends onshore. I was sure she would turn away, either from fear or lack of interest, but she swam closer and closer, until I could count her whiskers and make out the shape of her wet, feathery eyelashes. Her body bumped up against my legs. She wasn't forceful, but I could feel that she was strong. We probably should have been frightened, but neither of us was. We were just two wild creatures passing by on a wild morning, in a wild world.

Before swimming off, just as she came—wide-eyed and wondering—she looked up at me, as if to say, "Am I a mermaid too?" I looked at her, asking very nicely if I could please be a seal. She turned her body back out toward the bay and sank into the deep. I stayed in the water a little longer, but only because I'd been invited.

WILD, WILD WATER

There is nothing like wild water. It's primal, cleansing, and connecting. It always feels like an adventure. The variables are endless, impossible to imagine, let alone predict. Whether it's seals or snowstorms or a pocket of warm water mixed in with cold, every dip in nature seems to carry with it the promise of something unexpected. You can dunk in the wild Atlantic, your favorite bend in the river, a great lake, or your neighbor's pond (if she'll share it). Just be sure the water is safe, monitored for cleanliness and safe swimming conditions, and please don't go in the water alone.

My external watery world has taught me more about my internal world than anything else. There is no book that has delivered lessons as poetic or profound, no bike ride, no cross-country ski or hike that has stretched me in the same way the wild water has. The big lesson has been about control, embracing my humility and understanding that I am at the mercy of nature. I can check the temperature of the water, but I can't change it. I need to stay alert at all times, not just to what's happening inside my body but also to what's happening around it. Wild-water dipping requires a tough-to-crack combo of vigilant preparation and complete flexibility—strength, smarts, softness, and surrender. The wild water has taught me to surrender, and that surrender has shown me how to be free. I always imagine the water is hugging me, as if to say, "You are welcome here."

I began my practice in the Atlantic Ocean and I'm at home there. But I don't think wild water is for everyone. If you're looking for consistency, convenience, and control, you may find your wild practice extremely challenging. The water is dynamic and fluid, and that's exactly what it demands. If you're dead set on a 50°F dip at 7:00 A.M. on Tuesday that lasts exactly two minutes, it might be better to stick to the tank/tub; but if you're willing to expand your tolerance beyond temperature, to open up your sense of possibility (and freedom!), you will love it out here. I promise.

LESSON:

Wild Safety

Wild-water immersion is riskier than a tank, pool, or shower practice, but when performed thoughtfully, I believe it can be more enriching. There is a lot more planning that goes into a dip in the wild and, inevitably, a lot more pivoting too, but here are a few guiding principles I use to stay safe:

EYES ON THE SKY (AND THE SEA!): Mama Nature's itinerary might not align with yours. Be sure to keep an eye on the weather and never swim if there's a chance of storms or extreme cold. Be mindful of windchill and keep up with your water forecast too. Algal blooms, rip currents, pollutants, and wildlife activity can all impact the quality of your experience and safety. Check swim conditions before you dip and stay aware of your surroundings. If the water smells or looks different than usual, it's best to avoid it.

FEET ON THE GROUND: Sticking close to shore is safest. Keep your feet on the ground if at all possible. Even if you're a strong swimmer, your body may react differently in the wild water. You may tire more easily or find it harder to catch your breath. Open water often means obstructed visibility as well. Drop-offs may be sudden, and changes in currents and undertows may be tough to identify. Remember, life vests are always en vogue. And if you do dunk, consider wearing earplugs.

MATTER OVER MIND: I'm all about exploring boundaries and experimenting with an extra bag of ice in the tub, but the wild water isn't the best place to push your limits, especially in an emerging practice. Listen to yourself and listen to Mama Nature. If she says the water is 33 and you're used to 55, try easing into a lower temp in a more controlled environment first.

HAVE EACH OTHER'S BACKS: Never swim alone and, if possible, stick to designated, monitored areas. Check in with your people frequently and be sure to pack a fully loaded first aid kit, a charged phone, lots of warm clothes, and any safety gear specific to your environment (bug spray, bear spray, reef-safe sunscreen). Check the temperature of the water with a thermometer before dipping. And please, stick to the rivers and lakes that you're used to.

LEAVE NO TRACE: Be a good guest. Never approach wildlife or remove flora or fauna from the area. Watch where you step, watch where you swim, and pick up any litter you see along the way.

THE LAST DROP

You belong out there, in the open air, with all the weather and wildness and starlight and seals. You belong with salt sparkling on your skin, sand between your toes, and miraculous hair that don't ever care. You belong in the warm sun and cold water. The wild water is a study in surrender. It is giving up your bigness and bowing in your smallness to the magic of this world. Mama Nature will always be in the driver's seat, but she loves having passengers. Let go and enjoy the ride.

LESSON:

Wild Seasons

There is room for cold in every season, even—especially—in the warm ones. Now, for all our innovation, we aren't all that adaptable. At least, I'm not. With a little extra prep and maybe a shot of pep too, we can keep our practice going through the seasons. Here are a few things that may change as the environment does and a little nostalgia to help you embrace every little shift.

In Winter You May . . .

FEEL: Water and air temperatures can both be extreme. The water can be slow, dense, and syrupy. Getting out may be even harder than getting in so please take extra care. A warm bev and hot-water bottle in the car make a big difference afterward.

SEE: If your swimming hole is more of a skating rink, don't despair. I use a sledgehammer and auger to (carefully) break through the surface and create a shallow spot for dipping.

REMEMBER: snowflakes on your fingertips, flannel jams, pink cheeks.

In Spring You May...

FEEL: Snowmelts and rainy days can mean faster, stronger water, even flooding in some areas. Be mindful of changes in the current and exercise caution.

SEE: Just like land plants, water plants and plankton begin to blossom in spring. In the ocean, upwelling brings cool, nutrient-rich water to the surface; more light means more photosynthesis, and everything grows! Enjoy the springing of spring, but on your way to the water, keep an eye out for poison ivy. It loves the water as much as you do.

REMEMBER: daffodils, petrichor, big rubber boots.

In Summer You May...

FEEL: In July, your wild water might be more like bathwater. This can be frustrating, especially if you've gotten acclimated to a truly cold experience. Summer is a great time to explore new spots. Larger, deeper lakes and water at higher altitudes may have cooler temperatures.

SEE: Summer means early morning sunrise magic. Wake up with the birds and take your time.

REMEMBER: summer camp, blowing bubbles, wet ponytails.

In Fall You May . . .

FEEL: Mornings become crisp, dark, and moody, and while the water may still be retaining heat, the air can be quite cool. Getting out may become more of a challenge. It's a good idea to get in the habit of putting on dry clothes immediately after your dip. Invest in a fabulous changing coat (mine is a Voited) if you haven't yet.

SEE: Lake lovers may notice changes in the water as the temperature drops, winds pick up, and the water "turns over," moving nutrients from the bottom to the top. In the ocean, upwelling stops and, with less vegetation, the water may appear clearer. Fall foliage lovers, beware of slippery, mushy leaf goo onshore when you get in and out.

REMEMBER: stacks of firewood, good apples, wool socks.

You belong out there,
in the open air, with all the
weather and wildness and
starlight and seals.

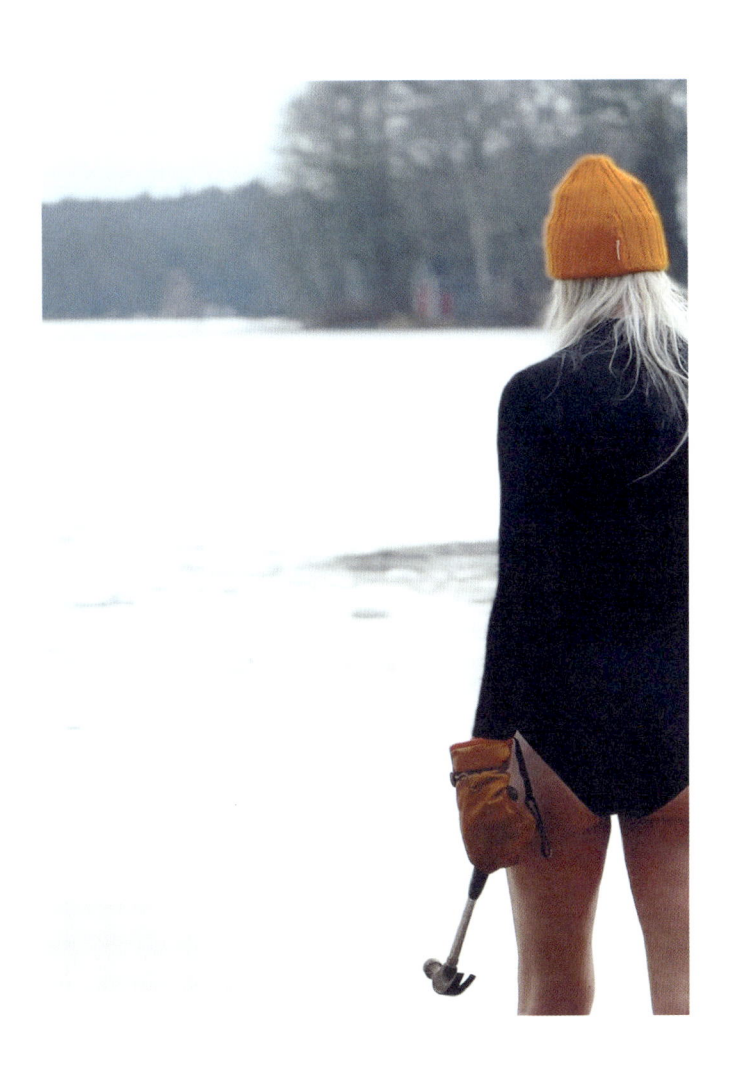

CHAPTER SEVEN

WELL-

BEING

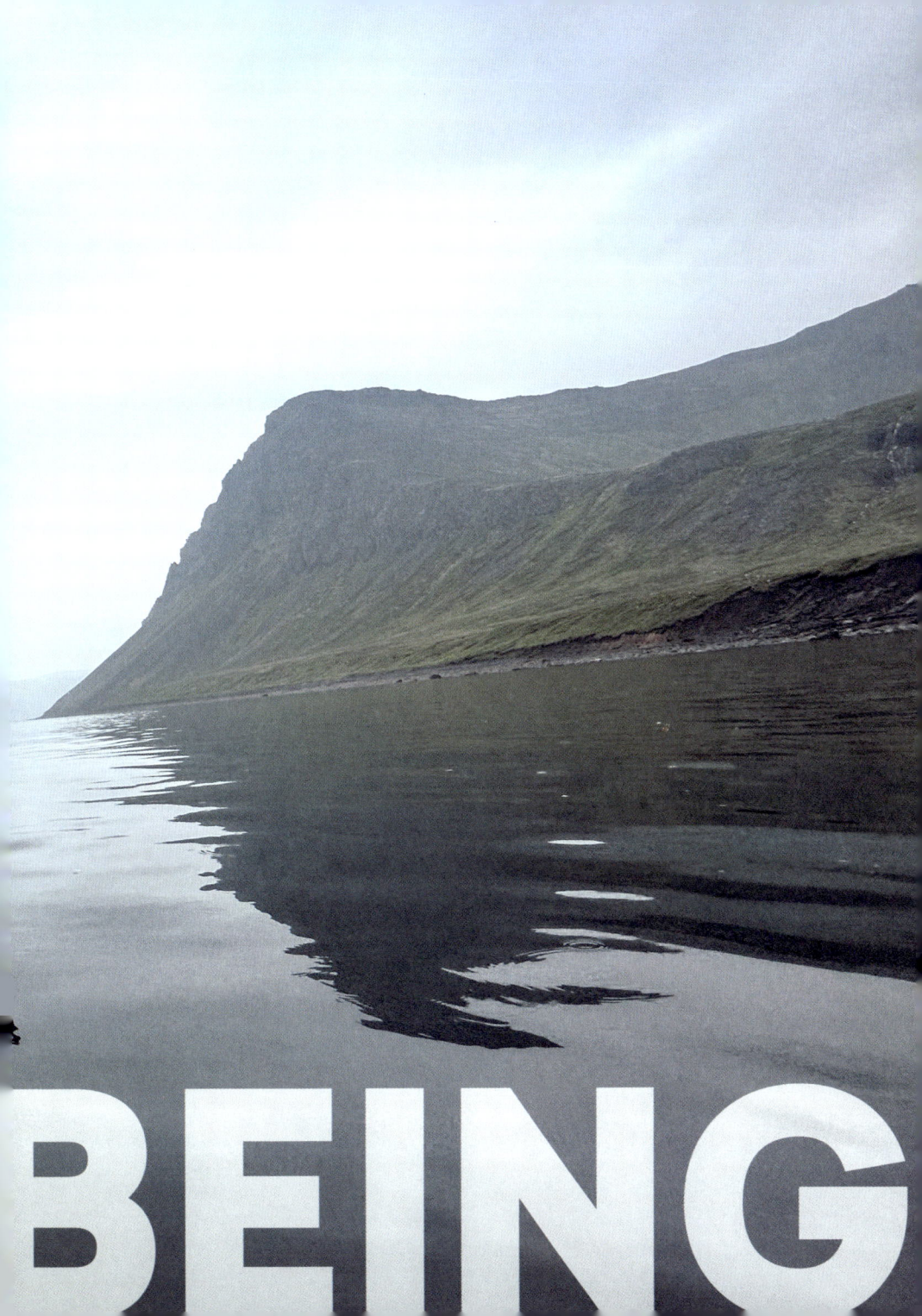

My relationship with the water began long before my cold exposure practice, but it was a different kind of relationship then, than it is now. In college, I was a rower. My day began just before dawn, in a moss and mildew-scented boathouse on the Connecticut River. The boathouse was always cold, lined with sleek shells and alive with the sound of sloshing water, brightened by the metal walls and roof.

Rowing is a challenging sport, a whole-body summoning that builds your mind and body into a fortress. There's ritual toughness to it—the early start, the rhythm, the constant feeling of pushing (and pulling) through. Catch, drive, finish, recover. Catch, drive, finish, recover. Some mornings, I would get out of the boat so sore that I struggled to stay awake in the afternoon. Carrying that feeling meant I was strong and safe and capable. We were taught to shut out the pain. The physical messages our body was sending us were to be muted if we were to go fast. To win.

Back then, I loved the water, but it was a strange love. At times, it was adversarial. More so than another team, the water was our opponent, the force to combat—waves, wind, chop. It was my mountain, the place I went to prove myself. I came to the river every day with discipline, focus, and ambition. If it was raining hard and filling up the footwells, we kept going. If there were waves splashing over the gunwales, we pushed on. If our fingers were blistered or frozen or both, we tightened our grip. Pain was part of our process. We looked to befriend it. I remember glancing at the water, dark and speckled with sun, and thinking, *not today, river,* as though it were egging me on just by shining.

In those days—even among elite athletes—there was little conversation about well-being. We talked about optimization and performance. We knew about our lats and our quads, the names of various useful regions of the spine, but we'd barely heard of the nervous system, and we'd never really considered the state of our mental health. The term "self-care" was decades from its first utterance, or at least decades until I was familiar with it. On the water, honoring a body meant pushing through whatever hurt: fatigue and cramps, stress, sadness, grief. It meant showing up for the team to do your part, no matter what, even if it resulted in not showing up for yourself. My body was a machine, an engine, a power source. I didn't really know it as a feeling body until I stopped being near the water, and went in.

My rowing ended after college, but the inertia kept me moving through the world like an athlete. I worked like an athlete and loved like an athlete, pushing, working, striving for excellence. I was working right up until March 2020. Even then, I was drawn to cold dipping for the physical challenge. I was fluent in the language of pain, challenge, and "not today" that seemed to come with the territory. The same energy I brought to the boathouse, I brought to the cold water.

When I ran into the water that first time though, my body (and mind) became still. I felt everything. It was arresting and scary and enlivening. I couldn't push through, and even if I could have, I wouldn't have wanted to because there was so much inside me, a secret universe of whispers and breaths and messages and new sensations that I'd conditioned myself to turn away from. There were sparks on the tips of my fingers and a fizzing all the way up my back. I had an ache in my elbows and a buzz in my temples. Then, peace all over, a luminous, kaleidoscopic star-scape of peace that shone from the inside out.

How had I never seen it before?!

How had I never felt it?!

I'd picked "strong" over everything else. And so, I made a promise to softness.

Dipping in the Merrimack River has given me my body back. It has shown me how to delight in it and listen to it. It has filled me up with gratitude for the gloriousness of aging, the waves of womanhood, and the wonder of being alive. Upriver, on any given morning, there is a team of young women doing pause drills and power 10s and seat racing, rowing their way another hundred meters and another. I picture them often. I root for them. Many miles away, just to the left of the ocean, I'm doing good work too, deconditioning, standing still in the water, in my body, in love. And finally, I'm winning.

HEALTH VERSUS WELL-BEING

Though cold dipping is a bit of a wellness wunderkind, data that captures its benefits is not yet consistent or extensive enough to say whether the practice is definitively healthy, or even safe. We do know it can be dangerous for some individuals. Like many things that become popular before proven, the practice has garnered warranted skepticism and, unfortunately, near-instant fad status. We don't have enough evidence about health impacts, especially long term, to back up the "miracle" claims many have made. This lack of evidence doesn't mean there isn't promising information emerging. It doesn't mean there isn't potential for cold dipping to improve health. It just means that, for now, the conversation about cold immersion is better centered around overall well-being than health.

I appreciate a scientific perspective. I'm a gobbler-upper of studies, but even my own data doesn't properly convey the relationship between cold-water immersion and wellness. Yes, I'm sleeping better. I don't get sick. I respond better to stress. But the biggest change for me has been my sense of embodiment. In the cold water, my body is adamant that I pay attention, that I feel breath moving through my nose and blood pooling in my cheeks, that I welcome each sense as it lights up in my consciousness—steam after a slow rain, the waking of the first birds, the glow of a juicy sensual moon. My success at the practice is completely dependent on my ability to listen to what my body tells me. And dipping has made me a better listener outside the water too. Every time I dip, I come home to myself, and to me, that sense of home *is* well-being. My body and mind are at ease. My heart is open. I'm grateful.

I urge my fellow dippers to really think about how the cold water makes them feel. It's a practice not a pill. Does the cold water make you more vibrant? Aware? Awake? Or does it make you feel anxious? Does it give you energy or take it away? Individual results can vary, so listening to your body (and your doctor's advice) is crucial.

There is much we don't know about cold dipping, but we do know that people have been practicing it for a very, very long time for health, social engagement, and cultural reasons. That history is significant. We know that its recent resurgence has created cold communities around the world, captivated journalists, and piqued the interest of doctors and scientists. What *I* know is that life is better for me when cold water is a part of my routine. It's the immeasurable things— the magic of my insides matching my outsides, the way I *feel* in my body—that tell me how "well" I really am.

Every time I dip, I come home to myself, and to me, that sense of home is well-being.
My body and mind are at ease.
My heart is open. I'm grateful.

LESSON:

The Skinny on Skinny-Dipping

I fell in love with my body in the water and I'm not alone. I can't count the number of women I've met through this practice who told me that, before cold dipping, they hadn't been in a bathing suit in years. Some were too uncomfortable with their thighs or arms or breasts or dimples to go swimming in their pools with families. I'm happy to report that most mermaids have found getting in the water together a life-changing recalibration of how they feel about their bodies.

Skinny-dipping is a silly and sexy self-love celebration that has brought so much joy to my life and my practice. While plenty of cultures embrace clothing-optional swimming, in America we're still trying to free the nipple, so stripping down requires a little extra prep. These are the bare-naked rules I live by:

RIGHT PLACE, RIGHT TIME: Unless you're on private property or in a designated nude swimming area (I love you, Baker Beach), skinny-dipping is illegal in the United States. So, scout your spot very carefully or, even better, make friends with someone who has private access to water. Be mindful of timing as well. You don't want to be getting out of the water midday, just as the local Boy Scout troop is rounding the corner.

NO PICTURES, PLEASE: Respect your fellow dippers' privacy. Be **in** the moment, don't document it. No pictures **at all**. Keep a phone handy for safety and absolutely nothing else.

SUNSCREEN EVERYTHING: Sun's out, buns out! Do not burn the buns. Be liberal with your reef-safe sunscreen.

NEVER SWIM ALONE: As tempting as it may be for bashful mermaids to keep their skinny-dip a secret, swimming alone, with or without a suit, is not safe. Bring a (bosom) buddy.

KEEP YOUR STUFF SECURE AND IN SIGHT: The only thing worse than chasing bra and underwear tumbleweed across a blustery beach completely naked is forgetting where you put them in the first place. Use a backpack or a rock to keep your clothing secure, and don't forget where you stash your stuff. I speak from experience.

THE LAST DROP

When I think of my body, I think "love." My hands are love and my bespectacled eyes are love, and my grey hair, especially my grey hair, is love. It's taken me many years and many dips to feel this all the way through. Cold exposure does what it promises. It unveils, unmasks, and, in many ways, unencumbers. Uniquely, the practice demands strength and softness, that we challenge our bodies and cherish them, every single time we're in the water. Every body is different but every body is love.

BODY OF WATER

Often, when I'm in the water and experiencing self-doubt or getting the sense that I'm somewhere I don't belong, I think about how much water there is in me. Our adult bodies are up to 60 percent water. Water helps us regulate temperature, dispose of waste, and carry oxygen all over our body. It's so much of us, it's almost hard to believe. Let's take a look!

Brain: 73 percent
Heart: 73 percent
Skin: 64 percent
Lungs: 83 percent
Muscle: 79 percent
Bone: 31 percent

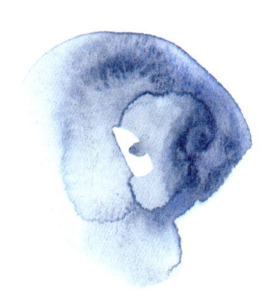

CHAPTER EIGHT

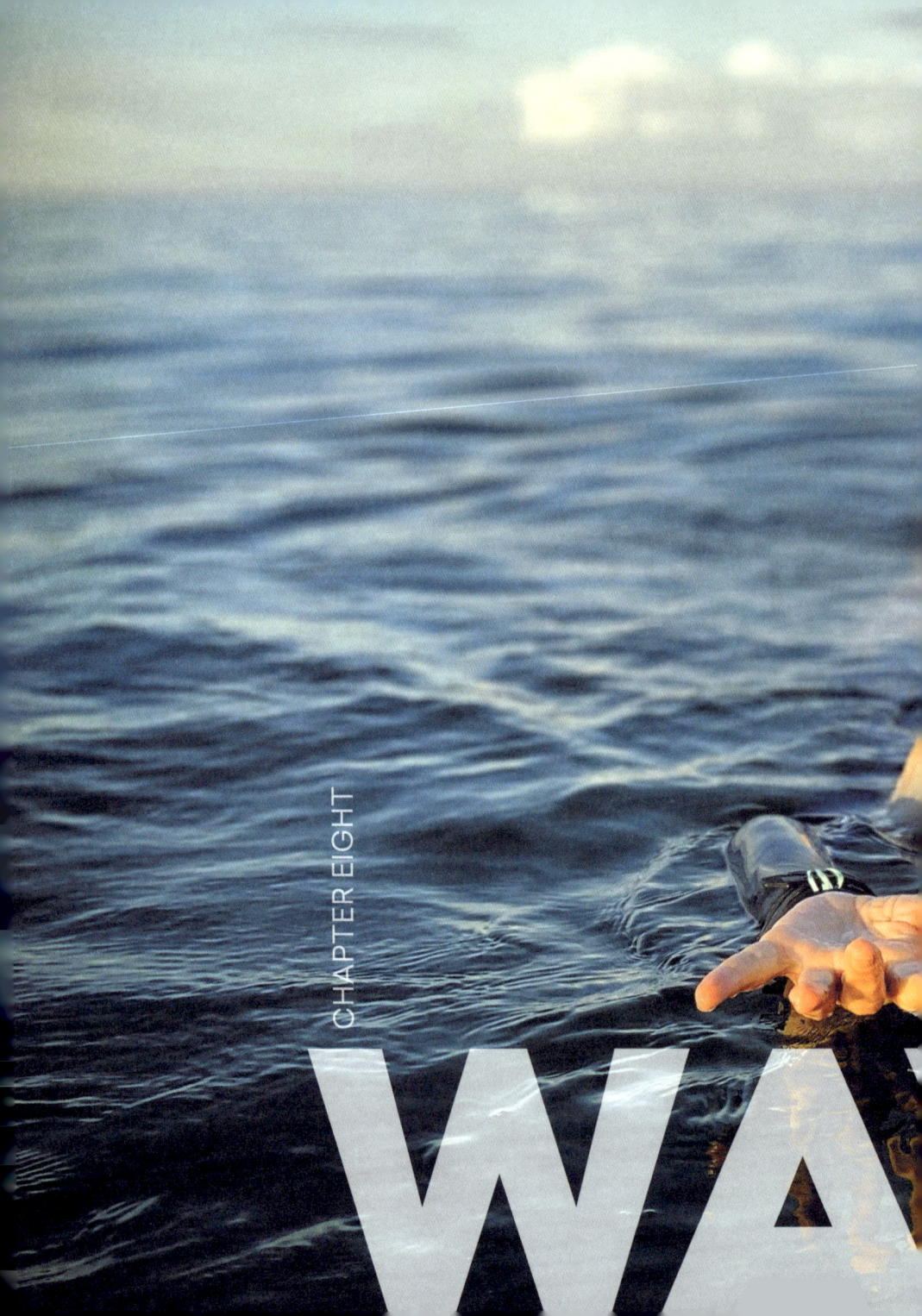

WA

VES

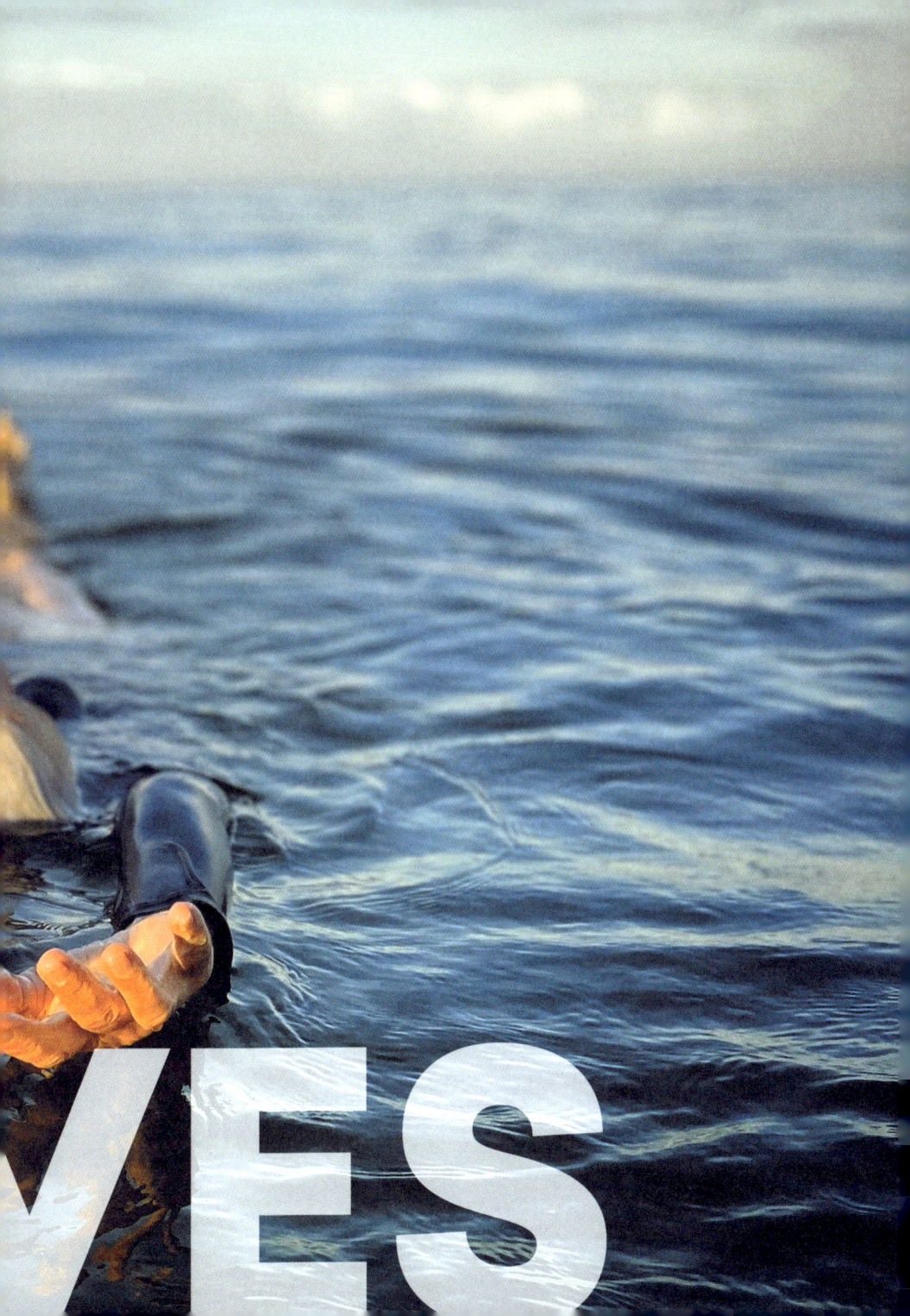

Not long ago, a little girl asked me if I'd ever seen a dragon. I said no, but quickly after, I realized I'd seen one just that morning. Around 6:00 A.M., it had been me, the sledgehammer, and the stock tank. A freezing, stinging rain pinched my cheeks and the battery on my headlamp was dying a slow, flickering death. I had to poke it back on every thirty to forty seconds. And it was hard, the kind that leaves a mark on your forehead.

I stood over the tank, looking down at the water. It was covered with ice, covered with snow. I wasn't sure how hard I wanted to work to do the work. There was no pressing conversation or reflection calling me to the water. I didn't have to do it—the most dangerous and alluring truth of any practice—and I didn't want to. I felt panicked by my boredom and baffled that my practice, which at one time had felt like a baptism, had become a routine, as spiritually significant as brushing my teeth or eating vegetables. I looked at the water and all I could think was *kale*.

And then, when I thought I couldn't be any less motivated, Ruby DeBina arrived. Ruby DeBina, the voice of resistance, not reason; Ruby DeBina, my inner kid sister, my evil(ish) alter ego, the reason this *do*er doesn't *do;* Ruby DeBina, mother of all dragons. Ruby was there when I was thirteen, telling me I was too tall for my platform shoes. She sat on my shoulder during the SATs and spent plenty of time in the boathouse, perched on the end of my oar. She was just one cubicle over at my first job and came in frequently from head office throughout my career. She was even there when my marriage ended. I don't dislike Ruby, necessarily, but I've never invited her over.

Ice clinking against the side of the tub, sun starting to rise, rain mercifully slowing, I moved closer to the water, grabbing the cold frozen metal edge and gathering my courage.

Why? Ruby asked.

I rifled through the answers and reasons, unable to find the perfect one. The lessons of the practice had leveled off. Getting in the water didn't feel particularly heroic anymore. When I thought about it—when *she* made me think about it—the practice felt pedestrian, un-sparkly, un-special.

Why? she asked again from the corner of my psyche, tapping away at a text message on her Ruby DeBina phone with her long Ruby DeBina nails, big wad of gum in her cheek. She looked bored, desperately so.

Steam swirled from my nostrils like chimney smoke and, finally, my headlamp died. I pressed the button a few times to be sure; *click, click, click,* dead, *click, click, click,* dead. I was getting cold too, and not good cold, tired cold. It's one thing to start your day with a few galvanizing minutes in the water and another to spend it standing in your swimsuit in the freezing rain in January, in Massachusetts, existentially tuckered out.

I can do this, I told myself.

It's not like it's hard, Ruby snapped back, crossing her arms, waiting on me to give in so she could get on with her day.

She was right. Getting in the water wasn't the challenge anymore. *She* was.

I kicked off my boots and winced as the soles of my feet hit the bristly, crunchy surface of the snow.

You don't have to do this, Ruby reminded me.

As the sky turned dusty pink, I settled into the icy tank. The water was shocking. My body was stiff. My lungs felt puny and my hands were gripping the sides of the tub, knuckles sharp-looking and white. There was a sobriety to the moment, a clarity, finally, quiet. Because Ruby DeBina wasn't there. Dragons don't like the water.

I closed my eyes. There was a cold whisper and it was mine: *You don't have to do this, but you can.*

COLD WALLS

Now and then, when I'm in the water with my mermaids, normally toward the end of a dip, someone will say, "Ooof. That last one. That was a big wall."

And we all know exactly what they're talking about.

Barriers come up. Resistance is real. It's easy to dip, walk, run, and meditate when we're on a mission, but when we're not, we have to choose our practice all over again. We call these moments of apathy, avoidance, or apprehension "cold walls." These are the challenges behind the challenge. When a practice progresses and getting in the cold water is no longer a physical contest, the spiritual contest begins.

Walls don't always look the same. Some days the wall might be getting up, out of bed, and finding your way to the water's edge. Other days, it might be getting out of the water (getting out is often the hardest part for me). The wall might be the weather. Against all odds (every single one of the odds!), I'm a complete sourpuss in the heat and, in the thick of July when I know the "cold" water in the Bay is hovering just below a balmy 60 degrees, it takes a lot to get me down to the beach. When I do get there, I can admit, I'm not that pleasant to be around. A wall can be who you're dipping with. Or, who you're not.

Clumsily, grumpily, and sometimes muttering, I've learned to approach resistance as its own joyful (and inevitable) immersion, to love it as an opportunity to get creative, honest, brave, and playful, to relish my time with dragoness Ruby DeBina, who, between her shrugs and eyerolls, always has something to teach me. If, over time, your practice gets harder, I hate to break it to you, but you're probably doing something right. The water isn't asking more of you, you're asking more of yourself.

Resistance is a reminder that a cold-water immersion, perhaps more than any other kind, is fluid. Dedication and determination to it come in waves, phases, and seasons and that's OK. We have to trust that, in the water, we'll find new questions and deeper truth, the patience to face our "dragons," and the curiosity to explore what's behind the wall.

LESSON:

Cold Windows

Walls are completely normal, but that doesn't make them fun. It's hard when something that used to light us up starts to feel like taking the trash out to the curb. I promise, it's not a forever feeling. I don't know any that are. As your practice progresses through the months and years, the water may demand less focus. You may get distracted more easily. Your practice may not feel as functional or physically rewarding as it once did. Sometimes, people even develop new fears (Oh no! It isn't working. Why isn't it working?! What's wrong with me?). Have compassion for yourself. Feel all the feels. But remember, cold ones, there's a perfect place in every cold wall for a window.

For me and many of my mermaids, barriers come up in three primary areas: internal, environmental, and existential. If physical walls such as pain, fatigue, or dizziness show up, it's best to press pause, rest, and maybe head to the doctor. But for mental issues, simple tweaks to your practice can lead to big shifts in perspective. Here are just a few examples:

Internal Walls

WALL: "I don't crave the water anymore." "What happened to the rush?" "Bored, bored, bored."

Over time, you **will** get used to getting cold because your body is a lovely, gloriously intelligent thing. You're likely still experiencing a cocktail of delicious endorphins with each dip, but as your practice deepens you build tolerance, and getting in may not pack the same punch that it used to.

WINDOW: First, congratulations! At some point, you probably thought you'd never be here, accustomed to doing something so hard, so capably and comfortably. Wow. Second, it's time to stop thinking of your practice as getting into the water, surviving the water. Think of it as getting into your body, into yourself. How calm can you get? How present can you be? How quiet? Focus on building those strengths.

Environmental Walls

WALL: "It's too hot to get cold." "Rain, rain, go away." "My wild area is too busy."

Our inner weather and outer weather don't always align, do they? It's very easy to take every rainy day as a sign from the universe to stay inside and snuggle up, and of course, there is nothing wrong with choosing cozy over cold sometimes. But it isn't the only choice.

WINDOW: As a wild water woman, I am also frequently at the mercy of Mama Nature. The invitation here is to get creative and stay flexible. I prefer a quick, more brisk dip, but when summer rolls around and the water warms up, I have to stay in longer to get to cold and even longer to get to calm. I also have to look at whether my obstacles are really obstacles, or just inconveniences. There was a time I never would have dipped in the rain. Now, as long as there's no lightning or flood risk, I welcome it. I LOVE it. There's something so elegant about the way the drops settle in and bloom on the water's surface. Schedule shifts can help too. If my wild water spot gets wildly popular, I go early or late. Delicious dawn dips mean waking with the world, watching it open its eyes. Slipping into the water under a full moon, my primal self rises, and I feel brilliantly alive.

Challenge yourself to change with the seasons. And remember, if you need it, your home practice (shower, tub, tank) will always be there for you.

Existential Walls

WALL: "I'm not learning anything." "Am I getting better?" "What's the point?"

My, oh my, do I feel this. And I mean **deeply**. A cold practice demands intense spiritual stamina, and there are going to be days (*lots* of days!) when it just isn't there. Deep breath, friend. When the sparkles start to fade, there is still so much beauty beneath them.

WINDOW: Lean in to the big, uncomfortable questions. You might want to let go of them, but hold on tighter. Be patient. And don't be afraid to talk it out. If you feel like you need a hand to hold, by all means, hold a hand. A cold-water community can help here. Remember, these hard questions are important too. Not knowing is where we learn from.

THE LAST DROP

I have lots of favorite Rumi-isms, but one of his greatest hits is this:

"Listen to the sound of the waves within you."

I have leaned on this wisdom with my full spiritual weight, my weariness and worry pressing into the words. For me, most often, the waves *are* coming from within. For reasons I rarely understand, I am generating doubt or fear or boredom, or a plate with a little bit of all of them. It can be frustrating and disappointing and *sad*. I get sad when this happens. Practice doesn't make perfect. It teaches patience. The cold water can teach us deep, enduring patience if we let it. Wait it out. Love the waves in you like you love the waves on the water. Watch them come and watch them go. They will go, I promise.

DIP TRIPS

Got a bathing suit? And a sense of adventure? Let's go! A dip trip can connect us with new people and places, and it always helps me reconnect with my love of the practice. If you're feeling weary, hit the road, and then hit the water. **Here's how I take my cold immersion on the go:**

ASK AROUND. Locals will likely have the best intel on the hottest (but coldest) water in town. They'll be able to fill you in on things like temperature, accessibility, and safety. You can call the parks department or seek the advice of a cold-immersion group in the area (search #coldexposure on Insta and let the DMs flow).

GET THE APPS. Wherever you are, it's always important to monitor water conditions, but it's extra important when you're somewhere unfamiliar. Algal blooms might look different. Rip currents may be more difficult to identify. My favorite apps for monitoring water conditions are NOAA Marine Weather, Tide Alert, and Swim Guide.

RESPECT LOCAL LAWS AND TRADITIONS. If you stumble upon a great spot, stop. Be sure you're allowed to swim before proceeding. If you're a wanderer of wide-open spaces like me, it can be difficult to tell where public land ends and private land begins. If you're on Indigenous land, be sure to contact the tribal office beforehand and ask if and where swimming is allowed.

JOIN IN! If there's a local cold-dipping community, reach out! Most groups are thrilled to host visitors. All you have to do is internet sleuth and ask. Just be sure to keep in touch with your new friends and return the favor when they're traveling through your neck of the woods.

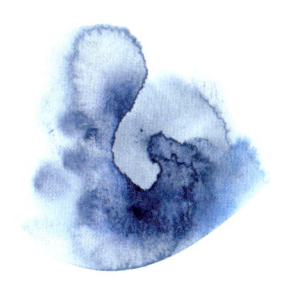

HOW TO TRAIN YOUR DRAGON

The best way to fight fire is with water, but positive self-talk helps too. This is what I tell myself when Ruby DeBina is in the water:

My body is a friend.

I belong in the water.

My heart is open.

If I am breathing, I am doing.

Be here now (thank you, Ram Dass!)

I trust myself; I love myself.

Let the water hug you.

Thankful, thankful, thankful.

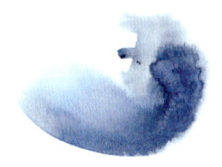

Practice doesn't make perfect. It teaches patience. The cold water can teach us deep, enduring patience if we let it.

WIS

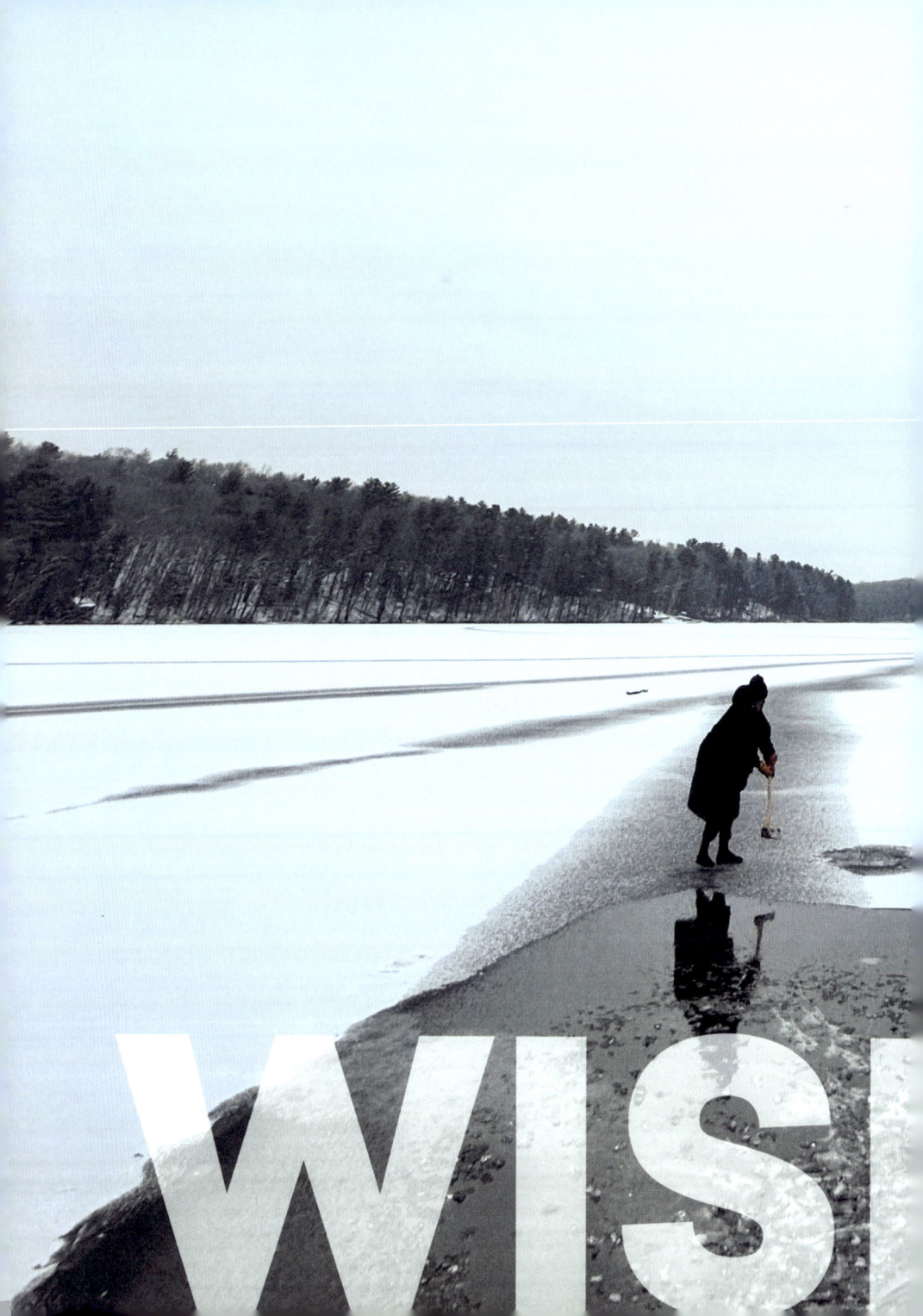

OOM CHAPTER NINE

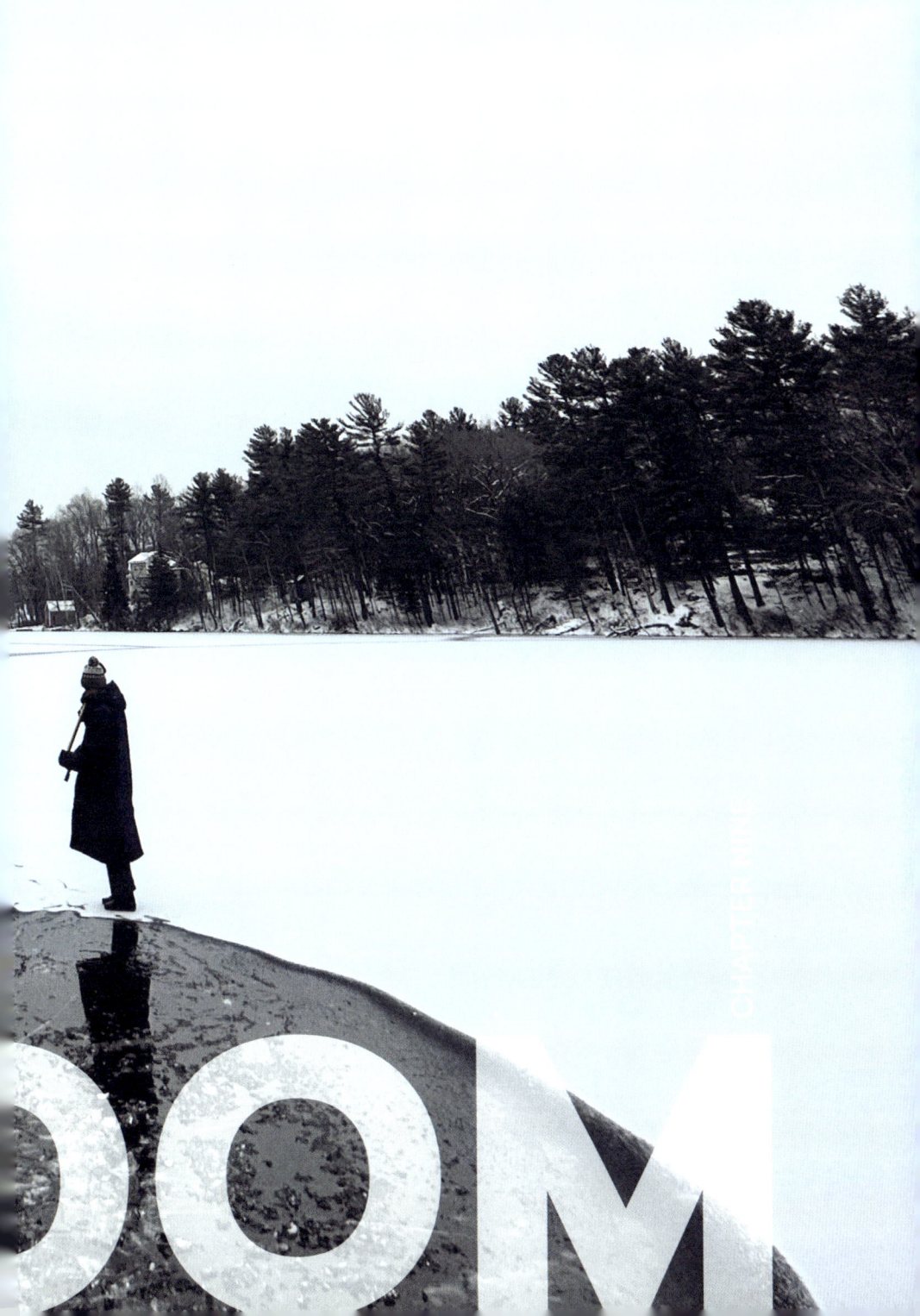

In December 2023, maybe an hour before sunrise, in the middle of a ferocious rain, I celebrated the third anniversary of my cold-exposure practice. I was in the tank singing a song about freedom by the earth-shatteringly talented Jon Batiste and I was feeling free too, watching the snow-sparkles dance in the glow of my headlamp, smiling at the playful shimmy in the stillness of winter.

Three years, I thought, *that's a relationship.*

After three years, you have trust. You've been there for some big life things. You've gotten used to the smell of each other's morning breath. You've learned to be patient among many, many other things. After three years, you *know*. At least you should know.

I watched the ice floating in thin panes across the water's surface and thought about what, aside from the happy-sad passage of time, I should be celebrating. I wasn't graduating into a phase of the practice. I hadn't won anything or even gotten markedly "better." I still had many days that felt like the first day all over again (actually, the third day—it was much, much harder than the first).

But shouldn't I know everything by now? I wondered. *Shouldn't I be wise?*

I took off my mittens and cupped the water in my hands. My mind wandered to the slice of celebratory cake I had waiting under a skin of waxed paper in the fridge, yellow sponge with chocolate ganache. I was not wise; I was still getting distracted.

Just then, a chickadee curled his black toes around the edge of the tank and looked at me, cocking his head sideways, as though evaluating the morning's fashion choice, a big woolly hat with furry pom-pom space buns. I looked back at his little Zorro mask (very fashionable) and considered for a moment my own mask.

Am I showing up to the water as my truest, unmasked self? Is any part of me pretending to be here?

My eyes fell to his variegated feathers, steel gray with thin strips of white and dust-bunny brown.

Am I seeing more? Noticing new things about the water?

The bird zipped off from the corner of the tank, his flight more buggy than birdy.

Am I doing it right? Am I flying too?

As I watched him pecking away at a too-hard safflower seed from the feeder, I realized that, after three years, still seeking, still learning, not knowing but chipping away was an accomplishment that felt so much bigger than the physical act of getting in the water. Sure, my body had changed. I hadn't had a runny nose in years, and I was no longer trapped in a cycle of "withstanding" the winter months. But those changes were insignificant compared to the shifts in my mind and spirit. The water had humbled me, made me into a student, a seeker, a person wise enough to ask all the questions.

Small floes of ice bumped against my body, and I thought about the miracle of every question that bubbled up to the surface. Three years ago, getting in the water was simply about getting in the water, and now, it was about bowing to the water. I had moved from tolerance to reverence. I was showing up to the water most days, and somewhere along the way, I'd started showing up to learn.

The water is where my soul is anchored. And really, that's all I ever needed to know.

WATER-WISE

I don't know if cold water makes us more intelligent. Maybe it sharpens our wit. Maybe we become more exact with our numbers and poetic with our words. Maybe we come up with more ideas, or better ones. What I do know is that cold exposure can deepen us, that it can be as much a spiritual or mindfulness practice as a physical one. In the simultaneous stirring of body, heart, and mind there is some kind of effervescent, synergetic, mind-expanding magic. For me, there is wisdom.

But what does it mean to be wise? And what makes the cold water such a uniquely enriching environment to learn? For many years, I thought of wisdom as the possession of knowledge, but I now see it more as the pursuit. We become wiser when our capacity to learn and our drive to do so grow, when we don't simply remember the words of a great thinker, but feel them resonating, shaking (or shivering) through our bones. In the cold water, we feel deep and think wide. We are still but stimulated. We are centered.

STILLNESS

I've talked quite a lot about how getting in the water sharpens my senses, a brightness shared, if not raved about, by mermaids across the globe. As one friend remarks, "The water does to me what I dream coffee will do." For me, this is certainly true. But the water can also calm us. Even being near it can help quiet and clear the mind.

A pair of recent studies by UC Davis, featured in a 2022 issue of *Journal of Environmental Psychology*, reported that viewing water (in comparison to a regular old patch of ground) may decrease blood pressure and heart rate and increase relaxation. A four-year-long European initiative called the Blue Health Project, aimed at increasing the access to blue (rather than green) spaces, offered similar insights. After the revitalization of a waterfront in Greece, citizens reported decreases in anxiety. Participants in Spain similarly reported increased well-being after taking walks of just twenty minutes in blue spaces. Whether our unique connection to the water is more cosmic or cognitive is, of course, subject to opinion, but our connection does seem to be strong and very much worth exploring.

When I'm in the water, after the initial shock, my mind and body become very still, a virtue all on its own in these furious, frenetic days. I'm able to better observe my environment and myself.

STIMULATION

Still does not mean uninspired. I do some of my best thinking when I'm standing in the Merrimack at dawn watching harbor seals at the edge of the cove or noticing that the honeysuckle has bloomed early. It's only because I'm still that I'm able to give my attention to these wonderful prompts. I'm not listening for the loudest sound or brightest color, but for the things that move me in a deeper way.

I'm also better able to give my attention to others, focusing more completely in conversations and, hopefully, contributing more thoughtfully. The group I dip with on the West Coast has turned into a bit of an open-water salon. We often decide on a topic before getting in the water, and once we're in, we discuss and debate until we're ready to get out.

CENTEREDNESS

Everybody's God is different, but mine can swim. When I'm in the water, I feel as though I'm in communication with her. From baptism to bathing in the Ganges to the four acts of wudu, water has long been tied across many cultures to ritual purification. And even among the most agnostic of us, there seems to be something innately cleansing and connecting about getting in the water.

So many of my fellow dippers echo this sentiment. My mindful mermaids liken the cold water to a meditation and my churchgoers compare it to Sunday service. While I'm not particularly religious, the time I dedicate to my cold dips feels holy. The water holds our entire history. It's my connection to both our past and future.

LESSON:

Water Types

Three years ago, all water was the same to me, but I know so much better now. I've been learning. Mostly, I've been learning to learn. Observing what kind of water I'm in helps me clear my mind and get still. It helps me to connect to my environment and keeps me centered when my mind starts to drift downriver. From this place, I do some of my very best reflecting. And you might too!

These are the waters I swim in:

SLOW WATER: Lazy, hazy, sloshy river perfection. I can see all the bits and pieces and stories floating by on the current. It reminds me to dial down the inner chaos and go with the flow.

SYRUPY WATER: The sticky stuff! Dark, inky, and sweet, this water clings to the rocks and my skin and refuses to dry. It invites me to think about where I'm "sticking." Am I fixated on a worry or facing resistance? Am I having trouble accepting something challenging? Am I being stubborn? (never!) These can be difficult reflections for me. Thankfully, sticky water gives the best hugs. Often sticky water is the coldest.

SPARKLY WATER: It's like swimming in a pot of gold! Glimmering and effervescent, sparkly water is bright, cold, energetic, and loves having its picture taken. Sparkly water delivers a big shining truth: There is magic everywhere we look, if we commit to the water.

SHARP WATER: Water that bites the whole damn time. Sometimes the feeling is more of a buzz or prickly, but it demands that you pay attention. This is water that wakes me up right away and helps me summon intense focus.

FAST WATER: Going, going, going, fast water is my favorite kind of music. I'm extra sure to make sure it isn't in too much of a rush for me to dip safely. Normally, if the water looks fast, it's moving even faster. Fast water reminds me that even though the river/ocean/creek is a dear friend, she always commands respect.

THE LAST DROP

Wisdom isn't about filling our head with facts; it's about making space for knowledge, leaning in to our humility, and learning to absorb the evergreen lessons that are waiting in the world, prickly and potent, all around us. Wisdom is the difference between going through the motions and living mindfully. The cold water has made me mindful. It has taught me to find quiet, observe, and absorb. It has inspired me to *listen* and *look,* two simple skills that have made me a deeper, kinder, wiser student in all of life's classrooms.

SMART WATER

So much ancient wisdom centers on lessons learned from the natural world. Let's keep learning. Here is some timeless wisdom from the water and some of her favorite students:

"I know the joy of fishes in the river through my own joy, as I go walking along the same river."
—Zhuangzi, Taoist philosopher,
   from *The Way of Zhuang Tzu*

"O wise man! Give your wealth to the worthy and never to others. The water of the sea received by the clouds is always sweet."
—Chanakya, Hindu philosopher

"No man ever steps in the same river twice, for it's not the same river and he's not the same man."
—Heraclitus, ancient Greek philosopher

"Dripping water hollows out stone, not through force but through persistence."
—Ovid, Roman poet

"As the water shapes itself to the vessel that contains it, so a wise man adapts himself to circumstances."
—Confucius, ancient Chinese philosopher

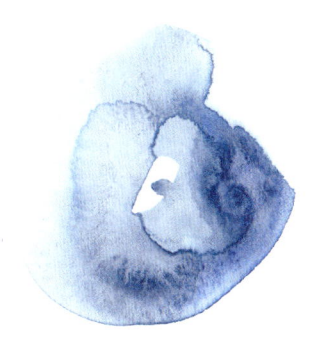

CHAPTER TEN

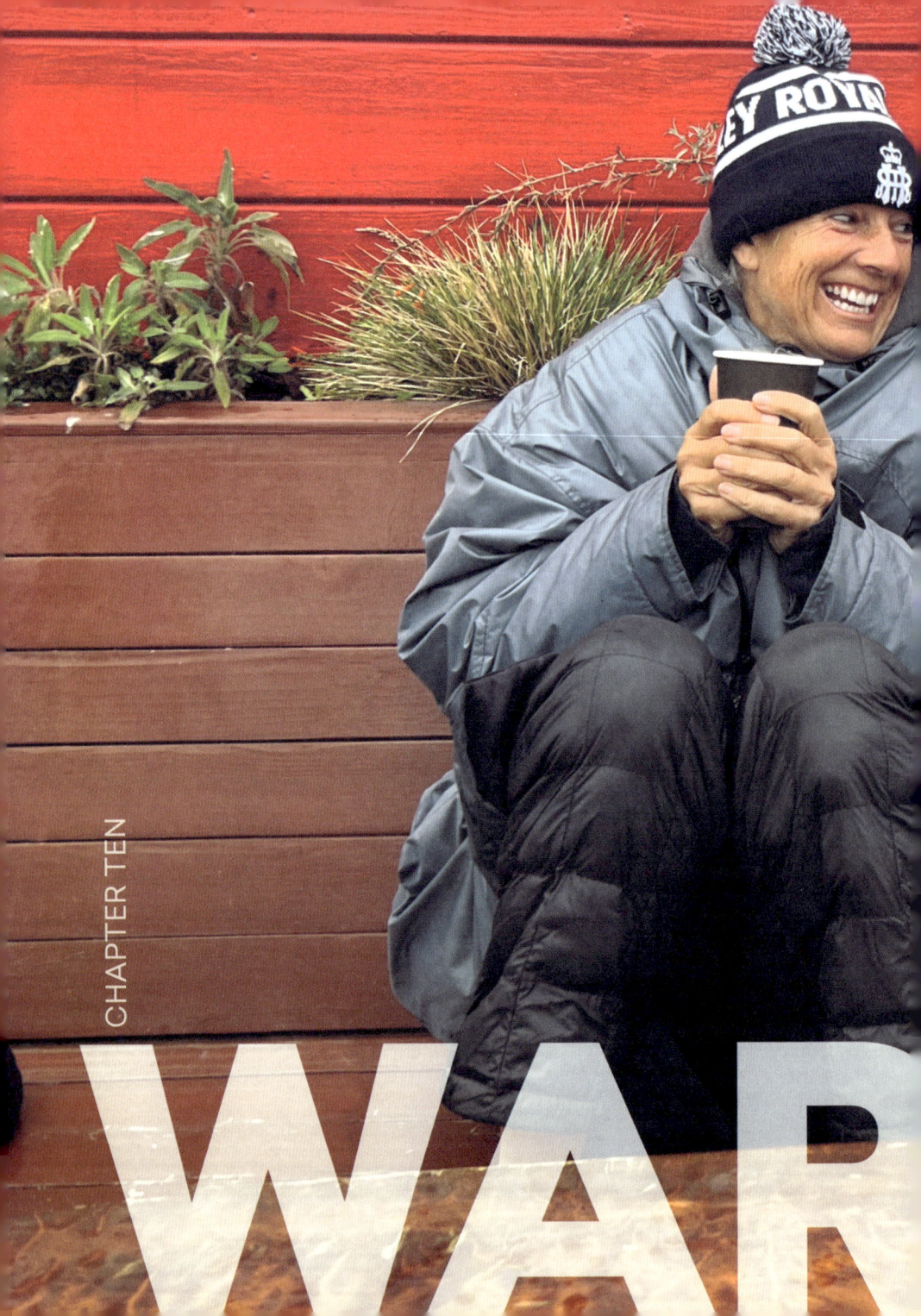

WAR

MTH

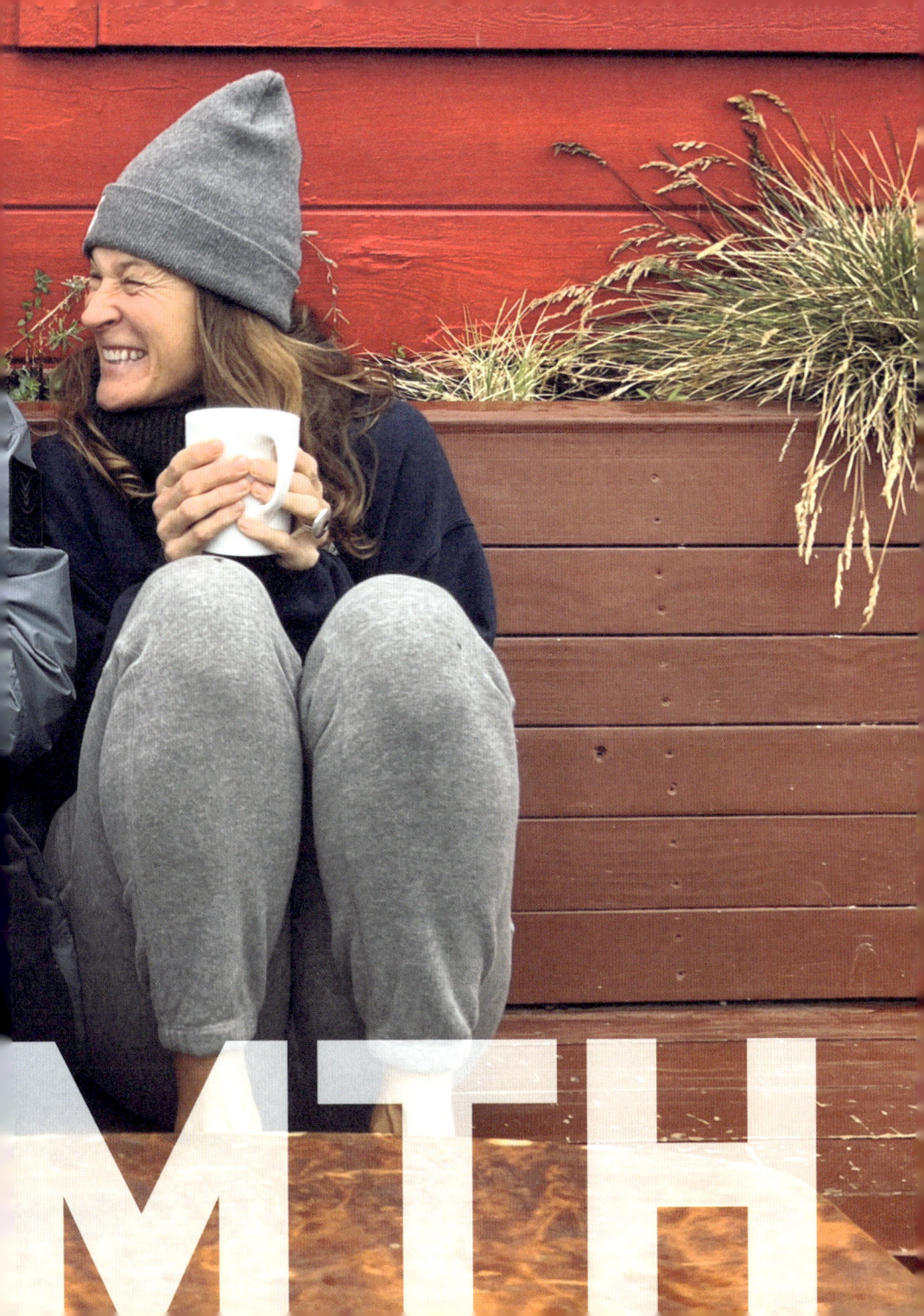

On the East Coast, there are mornings when the weather is scathing, the cold is so cold I worry about getting blisters from the air. I worry about the feeling of the water, the health of each one of my toes, the passing time. I worry about what I have done with my life and what I will do. I worry about everything. I worry that I can't do *it* anymore. *It* is mercurial, frequently morphing and shifting shape. Sometimes *it* is writing. Sometimes *it* is a relationship. Sometimes *it* is the dip itself, an act as familiar to me as my morning walk. I think about the cold water moving under the cold sky and I'm shaky-afraid. It's incredible the things a clever gust of wind can make you believe about yourself. Suddenly, there is doubt and the stories I tell myself grow teeth. The world darkens. The weather outside quickly becomes the weather inside. I can't get warm.

This first happened to me early on in my practice, among friends. I was at Plum Island, a place that seems to know me even better than I know it, a place that usually finds a way to say, "Good morning, Lib," in sunspots on the beach or with a Red-Breasted Nuthatch.

I drove up smiling for a dip one day with a golden-bright peace tucked somewhere perfect between my solar plexus and my heart. My darling mermaids, Ari, Meg, Sarah, and Claire were already there. I waved to them. I got my things together—changing coat, tea, towel, woolly clothes for after—and pulled my hat down on my head and opened the door.

A wind blew, the kind of salty stinging wind that shuts your eyes for you. Something happened to me. I knew it wasn't an especially nice day and had no intention of laying out on the beach with a novel after, but I hadn't expected the particular bite in the air. It took my breath away—a lovely sensation when you've planned for it, a disarming one when you haven't. When I opened my eyes, Plum Island wasn't as I'd left it in my mind. Sand that had once sparkled purple and bewitching felt peppery on my cheeks and legs. The wind was blowing, blowing, blowing, not a sea breeze or a storm, something different.

"Come on, love!" Sarah sang over the sound of the ocean, a roar that felt both loud *and* empty.

I made my way over to the mermaids. We didn't hug as we normally would have, and to this day I doubt any of us know why we didn't. There was a sense of urgency in that morning for all of us, indeterminate in origin.

Have you ever seen something that wasn't really there? I wanted to ask but didn't.

That's what worry is to me. And that's what cold is too, or what it used to be, uncertainty that has decided against possibility, a question that does more haunting than evoking wonder.

There was no sun in the sky, but we had to squint to protect our eyes from swirling microscopic debris. For that same reason, we weren't very chatty. No matter how well you brush, sandy teeth tend to stay sandy all day long. Wordlessly, we approached the water. I could feel the beach shifting underfoot. I could feel myself shifting too. In the long gray moments before we got in, my mind began rifling through worries: How would I get to the car after? Where had I put my booties? What if I got too cold? It was too cold?

But I wouldn't. Deep, deep down, I knew that. I looked at the water. While the rest of the world swirled, it smiled. I smiled back.

Instinctively, with my toes covered in surf, I grabbed Sarah's hand. And she grabbed back.

The water taught me how to do that, to reach beyond worry to trust, and hold it in the palm of my hand. The water taught me to be boldly afraid, so that I could experience bold love. It taught me how to be cold, so that I could learn how to get warm.

You got this, Sarah's grin said silently to me.

We walked into the Atlantic together and stayed together, not in the cold, beyond it. The sun never broke through, but I felt in a way as though I had. After the first aching seconds, my body started saying "you got this" and the water did too. My whole journey with this beach and this water had been scary and electrifying. It had been challenging and surprising. It had been emboldening and, suddenly, it was heartwarming.

Have you ever seen something that wasn't really there? I wanted to ask again, but again I didn't.

Because I knew the answer. Of course, it was love. The first dip is like falling in love. From there, the love grows deeper and deeper.

GETTING TO WARM

I crave a rush of cold water the way people crave heat from a hearth. The cold water is a cozy, light-filled home. A hug from my best friend. A conversation with my father. A walk with my boys. It's the feeling of trust, jazz piano, and loving-kindness. It makes me *glow*. I spent most of my life putting layers between my body and the cold, but the past few years have been dedicated to removing them.

It's no secret that "cold" cultures are also cozy cultures, experts at hygge, the Danish concept of creating warmth and contentment, feelings of pleasantness and safety in spite of (or because of) the bluster out the door. Learning to get warm, this has been the great lesson to me. I can't change the weather, but I can generate warmth and light. We all can. And when we do, the cold (or the dark, or the depth, or the fear) merely serves as a reminder to keep making more of what we need to keep warm.

LESSON: Get a Little Warmer

"Getting to warm" like "getting to calm" requires a certain, not always pleasant, understanding of its counterparts; in this case, we can call it the polar opposite. I talk often about letting the water hold us; getting to warm is almost like holding the water back, taking the cold, the uncomfortable thing, examining it, and finding a way to go deeper in, to get familiar, to love the unlovable. On particularly cold days (literal or figurative), this can feel impossible, but there are lots of things we can do to make those days a little warmer. These are things that help me:

HOLD A HAND: Is there anything better than holding hands? Walking into the water with someone is a loving act. It's emboldening, intimate, and deliciously cozy.

PREPARE PROPERLY: Proper prep is the best antidote to doubt. I might be cold, but my warm tea is in the car. It might be windy, but my towel is under the rock, it won't fly away. I might be nervous, but my dear friend is right here. Preparing is self-caring.

MAKE IT EASY: We know there are lots of ways to dip. Which setting feels the most like home? (Maybe it is home?!) Which barriers can you remove? If you don't want to drive or walk, it could be a good day to hit the shower or try the tank. On a day when I'm feeling nervous, nothing puts me at ease like Mama Nature.

SAY IT OUT LOUD: Be boldly afraid! Yell it! Declare it to the world! I love some positive self-talk, but I think a huge part of doing that right is doing it honestly. Having an ick day? Be icky, share it, don't carry the ick alone. I'll help you carry it.

LESSON: Understanding Afterdrop

Following cold stress (especially on a cold day), many people may experience a continued drop in core body temperature. This is known as "afterdrop." Your skin may warm quickly after a dip, but deeper tissues can take longer. Sometimes, after a winter dip, I'll get an unexpected shiver when I've been dry and onshore for twenty or thirty minutes. Afterdrop can be uncomfortable and, for some people, potentially dangerous. It's important to have a system in place for getting out of the water and getting warm efficiently, especially during the colder months.

Before You Dip

READY THE BEV: Before you leave the house, prep a hot tea, sipping broth, or other warm drink in an insulated cup to bring with you. Consuming something warm after your dip is not only peak coziness, but very helpful in bringing up your core temp.

SCOUT YOUR LOCATION: If you're not at home, find a good spot to get dressed BEFORE you dip. Be mindful of the wind (it can make the cold much colder!). If you drove to your location, have a dedicated spot for your keys. There's nothing worse than rifling through your stuff with frozen fingertips.

ORGANIZE: Know **exactly** where your things are. I love a familiar system. Pack them (and unpack) in the order needed. For me, this normally looks like laying out my bathmat and my booties beforehand and making sure my towel and changing coat are the first things I see when I unzip my bag after.

During the Dip

NOTICE THE TIME: Even if I'm in the middle of a winter wonderland fantasy dream dip, I'm mindful not to stay in too long. "Too long" can vary from person to person, but I err on the side of caution, always. Remember, your body may get colder after you're done. Getting out is harder than getting in. No one wins an award for staying in longer.

After the Dip

SPLASH WITH WARM WATER: Before I dry off, I like to rinse my feet and hands with warm water to help with circulation in my fingers and toes. I use an old water bottle, which I fill with hot water before leaving the house. It is usually just the right temperature by the time I get out of the water.

STEP ONTO A BATHMAT, DRY OFF IMMEDIATELY: You lose a lot of heat from your bare feet and, post-dip, the icy ground is not your friend. An old bathmat from home or the thrift shop will do just fine. Wrap up right away in your towel.

MOVE YOUR BODY: Jump around, dance, run in place, wiggle about, generate some personal heat.

PRESTO CHANGO: Invest in a roomy changing coat that covers your arse. Bring clothing that's easy to get into when wet (denim is a hard no) and layer with wool. Pocket heaters are great too!

GET OUT OF THE COLD QUICKLY: As much as we love mermaid love, you don't want to linger. Get out of the weather and into your heated home or car.

EAT SOMETHING: Energy out, energy in. Your body needs calories to keep warm, so not long after your dip, be sure to consume something nutrient-rich that really feels nourishing too. My go-to is warm scrambly eggs. Or cake, if at all possible :). I love cake. It's ridiculous.

THE LAST DROP

Cold Immersion not only tests our bodies and our minds, but our spirits too. Every dip, a question comes up: Can I do this? Yes, yes, I can. Knowing the answer to that question has brought me confidence, peace, and a wonderful feeling of warmth that I carry with me regardless of the weather. Yes, I can get in the water. Yes, I can care for myself. Yes, I trust myself.

Bafflingly, my greatest fear not only became my greatest joy, but also a genuine comfort. I turn to the water like a trusted friend, a beloved mantra, and the kind of memory that warms you from the tips of your toes to the ends of your eyelashes. Like magic, the cold water, ever-changing in every way, has become my solid ground.

WOOLIES AND WARMIES

Apart from a couple of items, chances are you already own much of what you need for winter dipping success. If you don't, I highly recommend thrifting before buying new. It's better for the planet and your penny collection.

Nice to Have:
HATS (one for in the water and a dry one for when you get out). If I dunk (you don't have to dunk) and then put my hat back on, I really want a dry one once I'm back in the car.

NECK GAITER. When my neck is warm, I feel warm.

MITTENS. You don't have to put your hands in the water, you can wear mittens, even while you are in the water. I often do! If you do want to put your hands in, use your underarms to keep them warm.

WOOLIES AND WARMIES cont'd

CLOSED-TOE SLIP-ON SHOES (not flip-flops). The easier the shoes are to get on, the better. Size up if you need to!

WOOL OR CASHMERE SWEATER. To put on immediately after your suit comes off. Material matters. I get all of my high-quality wool/cashmere from the thrift shop.

EASY-ON PANTS. No denim. No cotton. No elastic at the ankles.

WOOL KNEE-HIGHS. Surprise! They actually don't provide much warmth in the moment *but* they make it much easier to get neoprene booties on and off when you are working with ice.

CHANGING COAT/DRY ROBE. Get one that is roomy, easy to wiggle around in, and covers your arse.

NEOPRENE BOOTIES. Good for when the water is below 40 degrees and the beach is snowy or icy. Mine are second-hand neoprene booties with zipper up the side. Again, the easier on and off the better when it is below freezing everywhere.

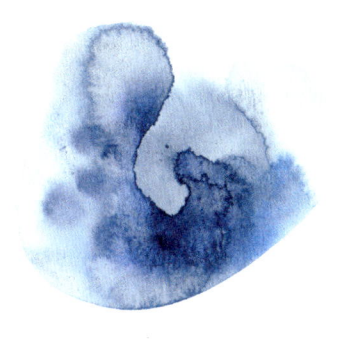

TALK COZY TO ME

One of the greatest lessons winter dipping teaches us is how to get warm. All around the world, but particularly in cold-weather cultures, there are wonderfully delicious words to convey that cozy, fireside feeling. These are some of the best:

HYGGE (Denmark): Pleasing contentedness, like a warm hearth in the winter

COORIE (Scotland): To cuddle, nestle, or embrace the pleasures in life

MYSA (Sweden): Snuggly feels, especially in the presence of others

GEMÜTLICHKEIT (Germany): A feeling of warmth, coziness, and all being well in the world

Learning to get warm, this has
been the great lesson to me.
I can't change the weather, but
I can generate warmth and light.
We all can.

REFLECTIONS

Water is one of the few things in the world that doesn't need testimonials. But when it comes to the *cold* water, we can be a little more wary. In case you need a little extra encouragement, my ever-generous, always-magical mermaids have been kind enough to share their personal stories with cold exposure to help you uncover yours.

"I first stepped into the cold Bay on the winter solstice of 2022. I finished cancer treatment in the spring of that year and the word 'aliveness' kept flaring up in my mind. I craved things and people that made me feel alive. I was terrified and thrilled on that December day as I gathered my towel, warm layers, and thermos of tea. I hired a babysitter for my daughter and was cagey about what I was doing because I didn't want anyone to know if I chickened out.

I did not chicken out.

I stepped into that cold wintery water and there was a churning, an exhilaration, a thrill, a dare. It remains all those things. The cycle of 'Holy sh**!' 'I can't do this,' 'I *am* doing this,' 'I am OK,' becomes a fortifying loop.

I sought aliveness and it delivers, every time."

—Kelly Wilkinson

"About a year and a half ago, I took my first 'dip' in cold water and I hate cold water. Born and raised in the South, I grew up being tolerant of the warm Atlantic of the Carolinas in the summer and later decided pools in Texas below 90 degrees could be a bit chilly. But people can change! And now I know cold water can change people. It's exhilarating of course, but I think it has become the most potent dose of 'everything is going to be OK' that I could give myself each day. And who doesn't like feeling that way?"

—Hilah Schutt

"I've been getting into cold water every Sunday at sunrise with a community of fellow dippers for just over a year. The first few times I drove to the Sausalito Bay in the dark hours of the morning, I felt like I was doing this totally crazy thing. But the deep pull to be in water and in community with a group of women was strong enough to get me out of bed. And then, the water changed me. I learned my own strength and joy and that trying new things is scary and hard and deeply rewarding. That if I can get into cold water on a winter morning, I can be a beginner and be scared in many other parts of my life. It feels amazing to be a beginner at forty and realize how many things I want to experience for the first time. How alive it makes me feel."

—Catherine Tai

"Why I decided to get in: I was moving through the most traumatic time of my life. My neighbor and close friend suggested I join her, to which I said, 'I don't need any more "hard" in my life,' but she said, 'trust me.' It was truly life-changing. That first cold hug brought me to literal tears. I was immediately hooked.

What keeps me coming back: Since then, my physical, mental, and emotional health have strengthened steadily. I have always had the most incredible family, friends, and community around me, but my mermaid family has added new and enlightened support and blessings in my life. We all have 'something' and dropping it off early in the cold water somehow makes anything and everything hard, easier."

—Devon McAllister Rothwell

"Cold water dippers are the best community. Rising early, stepping into the water isn't easy and yet it is a big remedy for my mind and body. Instantly all the worries and future thoughts dissolve as the water envelops my body. Focusing on my breathing and feeling alive becomes a meditation. Watching the sunrise or clouds shifting, reminds me of impermanence and the tidal quality of being human. This is an embodiment practice and I'm deeply grateful post dip."

—Bex Urban

"Cold exposure invites us into the parts of ourselves we have been avoiding . . . as humans we spend most of our lives hiding from the cold, protecting ourselves from it, and flat-out escaping it. To step into the cold water we start a dance with our fear and self-doubts, and to step into the water with those we love we allow our vulnerabilities to be laid bare. What a gift it is to meet ourselves more fully with a gentle hand to guide us through it."

—Breanne Burkard

"It was a rainy, windy day in November (a hurricane to be precise) when I first stepped into the icy ocean, clutching the hand of a stranger, another woman who was also taking her initial dip. That was almost three years ago and I've since been back to that cove—with that woman, who is now a dear friend—countless times.

It was post-pandemic and I was a newish mom in a newish town. I was feeling anxious, a little lonely, and altogether disconnected. I felt weighed down by the routines and ruminations and had refused any time to myself. When a new friend invited me for a swim with a group of women, I knew it was an opportunity I shouldn't ignore.

Swimming in the icy water at the mouth of the Merrimack River has rewilded me. A quiet and reflective predawn dip grounds me and prepares me for the day ahead. A boisterous plunge, hand-in-hand with my newfound cackling tribe of mermaids, reminds me that I'm worthy of genuine connection and laughter. The cold water of that cove continues to gift me presence and peace."

—Meg Connorton

RESOURCES

BOOKS

Harper, Mark. *Chill: The Cold Water Swim Cure*. San Francisco: Chronicle Prism, 2022.

Nichols, Wallace J. *Blue Mind: The Surprising Science That Shows How Being Near, In, On, or Under Water Can Make You Happier, Healthier, More Connected, and Better at What You Do*. London: Abacus Books, 2018.

Søberg, Susanna. *Winter Swimming: The Nordic Way Towards a Healthier and Happier Life*. London: Quercus Editions Limited, 2023.

Straub, Gale, Noël Russell, and Hailey Hirst. *Women and Water: Stories of Adventure, Self-Discovery, and Connection in and on the Water*. San Francisco: Chronicle Books, 2023.

Tsui, Bonnie. *Why We Swim*. Chapel Hill, NC: Algonquin Books, 2021.

FILMS

Body of Water
www.waterbear.com/watch/body-of-water

Chasing the Sublime
www.youtube.com/watch?v=wB3THSHPLuQ

I Swim
www.youtube.com/watch?v=OV2uRT4fTXA

Liminal
www.youtube.com/watch?v=StV7FGJtOow

Tonic of the Sea
www.youtube.com/watch?v=lvViuv0vIKU

INSTAGRAM FOLLOWS

@ebb.and.flow.collective
@ebb.and.flow.collective.sf
@redhotchillydippers
@whwolfpack
@northforkpolarbears
@coldplungecam
@thebluetits
@susanna_soeberg
@coldtitswarmhearts
@twomainemermaids

HASHTAG FOLLOWS

#coldexposure
#coldwatertherapy
#icefluencers
#wimhof
#vitaminsea
#wildwomanswimming
#wildswimmingspot
#wildmedicine
#soebergprinciple

ACKNOWLEDGMENTS

This book owes its existence to many, many people and many beautiful bodies of cold water.

I am grateful to W+O for their patience, kindness, and cheering from the sidelines.

I wouldn't be someone who could get into the ice-covered water without the unflinching love of the mermaids on both coasts. I love you. Thank you. #bestdipever

This book wouldn't have happened without the generous, original connection from Alex or the faithful, sparkling partnership with Shannon. Thank you.

I am also thankful for the guidance of my editor, Rachel, and designer, Vanessa. Their insight and belief in this book made it what it is.

Finally, to you the reader, thank you for taking the plunge.

CREDITS

All photographs copyright © Libby DeLana unless otherwise noted below.

Page 16: Photography copyright © Maaike Bernstrom/ MaaikeBernstrom.com/@Maaikephoto.

Page 25: Photography copyright © Annie Schweibinz/ @annie.schweibinz.

Pages 28–29: Photography copyright © Annie Schweibinz/ @annie.schweibinz.

Page 47: Photography copyright © Francisco Ureña/ SemperDrone.com.

Page 93: Photography copyright © Robin Lubbock/WBUR.

Pages 152–53: Photography copyright © Helen O'Shea of Ebb and Flow Collective SF.

ENDNOTES

Page 26: Reduce insulin resistance and boost insulin sensitivity, regulating blood sugar: Srámek, P., Simecková, M., Janský, L., Savlíková, J., & Vybíral, S. "Human Physiological Responses to Immersion into Water of Different Temperatures." *European Journal of Applied Physiology* 81.5 (2000), 436–442. https://doi.org/10.1007/s004210050065

Page 26: Activate brown adipose tissue (brown fat) and increase metabolism: Esperland, D., de Weerd, L., & Mercer, J. B. "Health Effects of Voluntary Exposure to Cold Water—A Continuing Subject of Debate." *International Journal of Circumpolar Health* 81.1 (2022), 2111789. https://doi.org/10.1080/22423982.2022.2111789

Page 26: Increase plasma noradrenaline concentrations by up to 530 percent and dopamine by 250 percent, improving cognitive function and mood: Berbée, J. F., Boon, M. R., Khedoe, P. P., Bartelt, A., Schlein, C., Worthmann, A., Kooijman, S., Hoeke, G., Mol, I. M., John, C., Jung, C., Vazirpanah, N., Brouwers, L. P., Gordts, P. L., Esko, J. D., Hiemstra, P. S., Havekes, L. M., Scheja, L., Heeren, J., & Rensen, P. C. "Brown Fat Activation Reduces Hypercholesterolaemia and Protects from Atherosclerosis Development." *Nature Communications* 6 (2015), 6356. https://doi.org/10.1038/ncomms7356

Page 26: Lower cortisol levels and decrease stress: Srámek, P., Simecková, M., Janský, L., Savlíková, J., & Vybíral, S. "Human Physiological Responses to Immersion into Water of Different Temperatures." *European Journal of Applied Physiology* 81.5 (2000), 436–442. https://doi.org/10.1007/s004210050065

Page 119: It's so much of us, it's almost hard to believe. Let's take a look!: Reed, E. L., Chapman, C. L., Whittman, E. K., Park, T. E., Larson, E. A., Kaiser, B. W., Comrada, L. N., Wiedenfeld Needham, K., Halliwill, J. R., & Minson, C. T. "Cardiovascular and Mood Responses to an Acute Bout of Cold Water Immersion." *Journal of Thermal Biology* 118 (2023), 103727. https://doi.org/10.1016/j.jtherbio.2023.103727

Page 144: A pair of recent studies by UC Davis, featured in a 2022 issue of Journal of Environmental Psychology, reported that viewing water (in comparison to a regular old patch of ground) may decrease blood pressure and heart rate and increase relaxation: Coss, Richard G., and Keller, Craig M. "Transient Decreases in Blood Pressure and Heart Rate with Increased Subjective Level of Relaxation while Viewing Water Compared with Adjacent Ground." *Journal of Environmental Psychology* 81 (2022), 101794. https://doi.org/10.1016/j.jenvp.2022.101794.

Page 144: A four-year-long European initiative called the Blue Health Project, aimed at increasing the access to blue (rather than green) spaces, offered similar insights. After the revitalization of a waterfront in Greece, citizens reported decreases in anxiety: Hall, K., Garrett, J. K., White, M. P., Grellier, J., Wuijts, S., Fleming, L. E. "Using Urban Blue Spaces to Benefit Population Health and Wellbeing." 2020. https://bluehealth2020.eu/wp/wp-content/uploads/2020/11/Read-about-the-benefits-of-blue-spaces_BlueHealth-Project_Horizon-2020.pdf

Page 144: Participants in Spain similarly reported increased well-being after taking walks of just twenty minutes in blue spaces: Vert, C., Gascon, M., Ranzani, O., et al. "Physical and Mental Health Effects of Repeated Short Walks in a Blue Space Environment: A Randomised Crossover Study." Environmental Research 188 (2020), 109812. https://doi.org/10.1016/j.envres.2020.109812

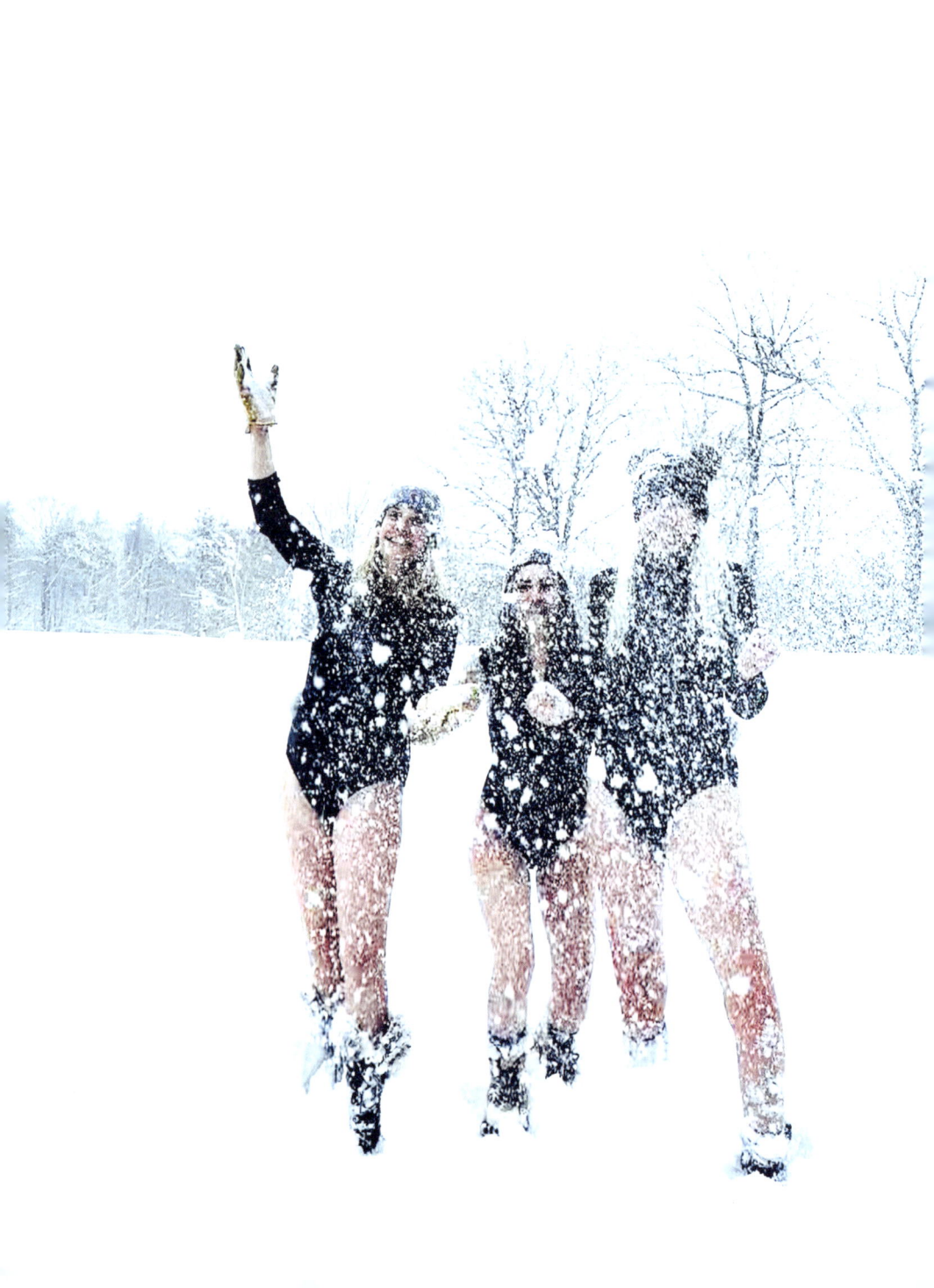